Natural Methods for Equine Health and Performance

Disclaimer

The information presented in *Natural Methods for Equine Health and Performance* is designed to enhance the reader's general knowledge of natural methods that are used in equine health. The book is intended as a background reference text only and not as a manual.

No responsibility can be accepted by the author, publishers, or distributors of the book for use of, or application of, the information provided.

The text is not designed to be used in place of veterinary care, nutritional expertise, or training methods offered by professionals.

Natural Methods for Equine Health and Performance

Second Edition

Mary Bromiley
FCSP
Chartered & Veterinary Physiotherapist

Illustrations and photographs by
Penelope Slattery

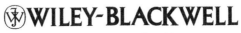

A John Wiley & Sons, Ltd., Publication

This edition first published 2009
First edition published 1994
© 2009, 1994 by Mary Bromiley

Blackwell Publishing was acquired by John Wiley & Sons in February 2007.
Blackwell's publishing programme has been merged with Wiley's global Scientific,
Technical, and Medical business to form Wiley-Blackwell.

Registered office
John Wiley & Sons Ltd, The Atrium, Southern Gate, Chichester, West Sussex,
PO19 8SQ, United Kingdom

Editorial offices
9600 Garsington Road, Oxford, OX4 2DQ, United Kingdom
2121 State Avenue, Ames, Iowa 50014-8300, USA

For details of our global editorial offices, for customer services and for information about how
to apply for permission to reuse the copyright material in this book please see our website at
www.wiley.com/wiley-blackwell.

Library of Congress Cataloging-in-Publication Data
Bromiley, Mary W.
  Natural methods for equine health and performance/Mary Bromiley; illustrations and photographs
by Penelope Slattery.
    p. cm.
  Includes bibliographical references and index.
  ISBN 978-1-4051-7929-4 (pbk. : alk. paper)   1. Horses–Health.   2. Horses–Nutrition.
3. Horses–Diseases–Alternative treatment.   4. Horses–Training.   I. Title.
  SF285.3.B75 2009
  636.1'083–dc22

                                                                                    2008030046

A catalogue record for this book is available from the British Library.

Set in 9.5/11.5pt Sabon by Graphicraft Limited, Hong Kong

1   2009

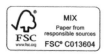

Contents

Foreword

Mary Bromiley is an incredibly talented chartered physiotherapist and horsewoman. She has ridden all her life, trained horses, and been involved in most equestrian disciplines, including race riding.

Mary comes from a culture and generation which, like myself, tends to 'say it as it is'. I believe one should consider Mary's concepts closely, I have often questioned her opinions, paused, thought long and hard and then reconsidered my position, as I have come to appreciate the decades of experience Mary has had in the world of the horse and the generosity with which she shares her knowledge.

Natural Methods for Equine Health and Performance is a precious resource for all of us that care for our horses. The text reaches out to help the reader understand how Mother Nature intended all animals, including ourselves, to deal with the challenges presented during our span of time on Earth. I find myself repeatedly thinking, 'that makes perfect sense' as I visit with Mary.

The ideas that Mary provides on these pages are priceless and to let them go without fair consideration would be a great mistake. Her concepts are of a no-nonsense nature and are based on the common-sense facts of a natural approach.

There was a time when I requested Mary to work on this old, beat-up body of mine and I believe I am better for it. It is, however, what I have learned from Mary about the ongoing maintenance of myself and my horses that I consider to be of the greatest importance. As a reader, you are blessed to have delivered to you the core principles of a very special and talented lady.

Monty Roberts
March 2008

Preface

The role of the horse has changed, becoming for many a recreational tool rather than, prior to mechanisation, a necessity. It is sobering to realise that only just over a hundred years ago it was quicker to travel from one end of London's Oxford Street to the other in a Hansom Cab than it is today by bus or taxi.

It is perhaps unfortunate that man has tended to humanise the horse, along with other species. Methods which have lasted since Xenophon (circa 371 BC) are suddenly not good enough, with the term natural horsemanship being adopted by some to embrace a new concept.

The cover picture shows a stallion, son of the famous Ben Faerie. He works as a stallion and performs a shepherding role on the Brendon Hills. His life is as natural as possible in a domestic situation, mimicking to a large extent the lives of horses living with nomadic peoples, performing useful tasks when required, otherwise living as nature intended horses should live.

Is it possible to apply natural horsemanship under modern conditions? What methods can the average, one-horse owner adopt for horse care in the twenty-first century in order to achieve a standard of excellence and avoiding methods which are regarded by some as abuse?

Ownership of anything, be it alive or man made requires information and understanding. Learning only from a book is inadequate. Observation, hands-on experience and, unfortunately, a degree of experimentation are required to become proficient. If illustration of this is required think of all the books on cookery. The recipe is there, followed to the letter by the budding chef, does the end result always resemble the picture? You are quite lucky if it does. With living objects this is even more apparent. How many parents have read the books on childcare, cover to cover, before their child arrives; when it does arrive, does the child conform? Rarely!

Ownership of a horse requires knowledge and the appreciation of the indisputable fact that centuries of domestication have not changed the natural instincts of the animal. The horse does not have a brain like man, see like man, or learn like man, and, unlike man the horse is ready to get up and run within minutes of birth.

Before attempting anything new perhaps one of the most important points is to learn enough to appreciate what you do not know. Everyone needs sufficient information to appreciate that which they do not know, in order to search for the information required to learn/be taught what they need to know.

This book attempts to give the reader, in a concise manner, an overview of the horse with emphasis directed towards recreating an approach which is as natural for the horse as is possible in the twenty-first century.

Mary Bromiley,
Exmoor, Turks & Caicos Islands

Dedication

This book is dedicated to the memory of the late Richard Miles, of Blackwell Publishing, editor extraordinaire, without whose unending faith over the years, I would never, after my first book, ever have put pen to paper again.

Acknowledgements

No book is ever written without help. The help I have been given has, as always, been exceptional. Amongst the many I would particularly like to thank are my grandsons, Mathew and Tom Slattery, who have with unfailing good nature, unscrambled my computer muddles.

I am indebted to my eldest daughter Penelope for both photography and drawings; my younger daughter, Rabbit, for doing my work on the farm to give me time to write; Sam and Camille Slattery, whose pad in the Turks and Caicos Islands is an ideal place to hole up and write; Nick and Sarah Slattery who have supported me through the writing process.

Part I

The Horse

1 What Is Natural Horsemanship?

Look up the adjective *natural* in the Chambers paperback dictionary and you will find two inches of text, leading you from pertaining to, produced by, according to nature, and on through a variety of definitions ending with illegitimate! The definition of the word natural for this text is *according to nature*.

For those people who wish to adopt a natural approach to horsemanship, the owner's requirements of the horse need to be considered. What do you expect from your horse? Do you wish to compete, and if so, at what level? The demands of top competition are now such that to win, athletes, unfortunately, need to manipulate their physical abilities often using substances which enhance their performance. Your naturally kept horse will undoubtedly be healthy and happy but is unlikely to win at Badminton or Olympia as natural living does not demand performance to those levels. If you are content to work and live with a horse, appreciating that there will be performance limits, then it is to be hoped that both you and your horse will have a lot of fun, enjoying life and companionship by behaving as nature intended rather than as man has demanded.

What do we mean if we endeavour to employ *natural* methods, remembering it is not just training we should consider, but also horse husbandry and the general, overall care of the horse including diet and living conditions. Is it possible to fully embrace *natural* in the true sense of the word, or is it best to take currently available information on horses living in natural circumstances (Fig. 1.1), the feral and remaining wild horses, as well as from archeological investigation and adapt it as far as possible to twenty-first century living conditions?

Unfortunately, no one knows the exact dietary requirements of the horse. Archaeology has traced the migrations of the various breeds and it appears that over the millennia various adaptations have taken place in the horse. Just as the kidneys of the camel have evolved to allow it to drink highly salted water, the Shetland pony living in its natural island environment and described in one book as being 'able to carry a man and his wife eight miles out in a day and eight miles back', can thrive on a seaweed diet. Other breeds would die rapidly if this were the only food on offer. One of the most important considerations of natural horsemanship is diet – 'what you do not put in you do not get out'.

Consider the following features available to a horse living in natural conditions:

- Eating a variety of herbage growing in soil uncontaminated by chemicals designed by humans.
- Sourcing and drinking fresh water, unpolluted by additives such as fluoride.
- Enjoying almost unlimited space and herd companionship.
- Living without rugs.
- Living without stable shelter.

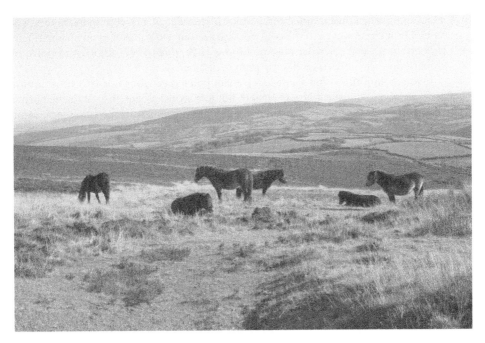

Fig. 1.1 Natural living conditions are still enjoyed by the Exmoor pony.

If we then return to the dictionary definition of natural, *according to nature*, it rapidly becomes obvious, that it is almost impossible in the twenty-first century to re-establish the completely natural environment of the original horse; pollution, the human population explosion, modern, intensive farming methods, the loss of old pastures, and the arrival of motorised transport are all cogs in the wheel of failure.

The time when the horse lived in large family groups, roamed vast tracts of the world, moving not only in tune with the seasons, but also in search of better forage, to replace minerals, finding these in certain rock outcrops, and to find fresh water, has long past. Even in places like Mongolia, where, until very recently the herds moved with the human family groups, the quad bike has appeared and in addition, climatic changes have resulted in sand storms burying vast areas of previously grazed areas. The last refuges of natural horsemen, in the true sense, have all but disappeared.

While the exponents of natural horsemanship should not be criticised, those purporting to embrace the art should remember that they are a long way from their natural beginnings. Man no longer uses many of the senses with which the species *homo sapiens* is naturally endowed. In reality, these senses are not lost but they are underdeveloped, for civilisation has led to us no longer needing acute hearing, in-depth observation, a well-developed sense of smell, intuitive responses, recognition of danger signals, natural balance, or the ability to seek missing nutrients by instinct. All these are still present and in people under the umbrella term 'Developing, or Third, World' they are necessary for survival.

In the general human population most senses appear blunted, particularly those involved in self-preservation. This is well illustrated by the high number of rescues, published annually, both on land and at sea, which suggests that responsibility for personal safety was apparently absent in many instances. People are apparently no longer able to sense danger, seemingly unable to read the signs of the approach of adverse weather from the sky, sense the state of the tide from sea movement, often setting off to climb up a mountain when mist is apparent, paddle on the edge of a river in spate, take a boat out, let children chase waves to the edge of a sea wall in a storm, swim on an ebb tide with a rip current present, or when the situation is such, due to prevailing conditions, that to embark on such activities is likely to end in disaster.

If you are not tuned in to nature, how can you expect your horse to react naturally in response to your wishes? Not only that, but in a world where 'instant' is the norm it can be hard to understand that becoming a natural horseman in the true sense, cannot be achieved in a weekend or by following instructions on a DVD, it takes years of interaction with the species.

Although horsemanship within the twenty-first century is still practised under natural conditions in remote areas of the world such as Mongolia, Turkestan and the Sahara, the local lifestyle of both people and animals in these areas is foreign to the average Westerner. It would be impossible to adopt the methods of natural horsemanship practised by the nomadic peoples of these regions, they would not fit within the living conditions enjoyed by the average Western horse owner.

The Native Americans were some of the most skillful horsemen in history probably because they viewed members of the animal kingdom as their relations and cultivated empathy between themselves and the animals with whom they shared the land in which they lived. The cowboy eventually replaced the Native Americans as the dominant force in North American horsemanship. Because the lifestyle of the modern cowboy does, to a degree, relate to present day 'civilised' living, there is acceptance of the philosophy of the greatest exponent of the art of natural horsemanship, Monty Roberts.

Monty Roberts was one of the first people to relate to the wild mustang and appreciate methods of horsemanship handed down through centuries of Native American culture. He will readily agree that his methods are not new, but rather an adaptation of the methods used for horse husbandry by the North American Indian after the return of the horse to the continent by the Spanish, following the invasion of Mexico by Cortes in 1520.

Monty is not in the first flush of youth and he is the first to emphasise that it has taken nearly 40 years for his suggestions to be accepted by the traditionalists. Having lived, for a variety of reasons, for a considerable time amongst the wild mustang, he was sharp enough to learn from his experiences and to establish the fact that the horse does not think like man, and that in order to interact with a horse man must respect and appreciate the horse's approach both to living with, and interacting with, other species. If there is another hidden secret to his successes, and it may be that this has not been emphasised sufficiently, or indeed even recognised, it is that the methods he employs when teaching, awaken and hone previously submerged, instinctive behaviour *in his human students*, ensuring improved interaction between handler and horse.

Unfortunately few horse owners wishing to be natural horsemen have the time to live in a situation which allows continuous interaction with their animals, and the horse is required to fit in with work, family and social life. This situation can prove difficult for the horse as their inherited instinct is to be part of a family group.

In some handlers mistakes arise from the perception that every horse will automatically respond in a similar manner if exposed to similar methods. This is an incorrect assumption; every horse is an individual and learning to identify the traits of each horse is one of the fascinating features of horsemanship.

2 Understanding The Horse

The horse belongs to the group of animals which provided food for other species, along with deer, cattle and goats. These are all classified as a hunted or *prey* species. Man belongs to the hunting group, the *predator* lineage, along with the big cat family, such as lions and tigers, and the dog family, e.g. wolves and hyenas; all of these eat the prey families. With this in mind and despite centuries of domestication, the horse still retains its survival instincts – rapid detection of danger, defence and flight. Any or all of these reactions can kick in within seconds if a horse feels threatened.

It is a good idea to consider horse culture before trying to interact with this species, and it is also important to appreciate that training/taming methods described as 'natural' are not, in the true sense, natural, when compared to the behaviour of the horse in nature.

The natural horse:

- lives in a family group;
- recognises and respects the group leader;
- communicates within the group;
- forms long-term social bonds;
- is able to select the herbage it requires;
- eats and drinks with the head down;
- drinks fresh stream or river water;
- uses the hairs of coat, mane and tail to inform the body of climatic conditions;
- uses the whiskers over the eyes and on the muzzle to provide spatial information;
- moves to find what it wants, following known routes like elephant families;
- does not wear tack;
- does not run in circles;
- does not carry a predator on its back without, in the early stages of this man-ordained situation, trying to rid itself of the burden.

How many of these natural behaviours do we interfere with? Which of them can we avoid changing? Which can we replicate or harness to the advantage of both horse and rider?

The domesticated horse (italics suggest solutions):

- often lives in isolation. *Allow companionship.*
- needs to learn to recognise and respect the human in charge, as 'herd' leader. *Employ this requirement.*
- cannot communicate as it would in its natural state. *May become frustrated at handler's inability to understand.*
- takes time to form a relationship with another species, such as man. *Remember, never be in a hurry.*
- is forced to eat what is provided, no choice. *Offer varied diet.*
- often has its food and water offered above the ground, e.g.: hay net, manger. *Replicate natural ground feeding.*

- is offered water that is generally polluted by chemicals, which are often alien to the digestive system of the horse. *Allow the horse to drink from fresh running streams if available. Test piped water supply.*
- is sprayed with show sheen and other sprays which insulate its body hair from the external environment, closing off a vital message system. *This is interference, do not use these products.*
- has its whiskers trimmed or cut off. As a result, the horse is no longer able to tell if there is sufficient space for its head. *Interference, do not cut or trim whiskers.*
- is unable to move to a fresh area if ground polluted. *Change pasture frequently, graze in rotation with sheep or cattle. Test soil for chemical lack or imbalance. Adjust if required using appropriate top dressing.*
- has a bit pressing on a sensitive area of gum, has pressure over flight/fight reflex areas behind the ears, also on belly (girth) and over reflex areas of the back if the saddle slips back or does not fit. *Use a hackamore or the bitless bridle and a saddle with large underpanels to distribute weight. Use natural material for saddle cloth, linen, cotton, wool, Navajo blanket.*
- does not naturally run in a tight circle, it has no need to do this. The co-ordination required to stay upright, in balance, carrying a moveable weight (rider) on a circle is unimaginable. *Reduce/avoid lungeing. Do not start circle work until the horse has learned to balance on a curve.*
- instinctively, the horse may try to rid itself of weight on the back, as for the horse this represents a predator attack. *Take great care when mounting, mounting block always preferable.*

Survival reflexes (see Fig. 2.1)

It is essential to appreciate that the wish to remain alive in the situation of attack by a predator has endowed the horse with *survival reactions* beside flight; *these remain despite domestication.* The horse retains *three areas* tuned for rapid reaction, designed to help survival when under attack.

- The first of the three areas is on the back. A predator runs beside the horse and attempts to mount the animal and bring it down by landing on the back, approximately in the area covered in the ridden horse by the cantle or back end of the saddle. Survival reflexes in this area cause the horse to hollow the back prior to bucking violently. It is very important to appreciate that these reflexes remain even after training. If the rider lands heavily on the back of the saddle, sits too far back or the bareback rider is thrown too far backward, the horse will first tense the back, then hollow, although when trained and accustomed to weight on the back, it may not buck.
  A tense, hollow back can be damaged by rider weight and it is this posture which is the primary cause of many back problems. In addition, with the back incorrectly positioned, the horse is unable to move in an easy, fluid manner.
- The second attack point is the poll. The predator attempts to break the neck of its prey where the head joins the neck. The reaction of the horse to sudden discomfort behind the ears is to throw its head violently upward. Minimal discomfort, often caused by an ill-fitted head piece, and/or a brow band that is too tight, can trigger these survival reactions and may even cause head shaking. The trained horse, doing its best to comply with rider requests, and stimulation of reflex actions, over which it has no control, are causing the head shake.
  In 1998, Dr. Cook, of the USA, designed the cross-under, bitless bridle. The principle behind the design relied on subtle changes in head position, making use of reflex

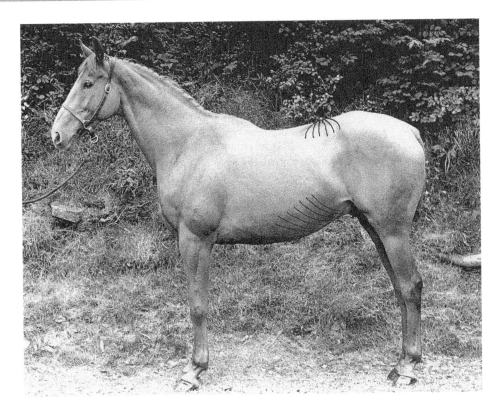

Fig. 2.1 Survival reflex areas.

points for control. This new bridle was said to be the first advance in the technology of communication between horse and rider for 6000 years. Martin Pipe, champion trainer for 15 years, was never averse to new innovations. Tony McCoy, champion steeplechase jockey agreed to ride a horse, wearing the bridle, in an NH race; interestingly the horse won by 9 lengths. Unfortunately riding without a bit is, in some instances, considered unethical and the subject is under currently review by the Veterinary Committee of the Jockey Club, UK.

- The third reflex area is located on the underside of the belly, and backward to teats or sheath. The horse tries to avoid having its belly ripped open by the predator; stimulation of these reflex areas may result in the horse lashing out. Your horse is not being badly behaved when it apparently tries to kick whoever is grooming or washing these areas; once again, natural survival reflexes have taken over behaviour.

Wild horses roam over and enjoy thousands of acres, travelling up to thirty miles a day. Domesticated horses with adequate space may not feel as threatened when early interaction with man begins as those confined to a small area, and although the two exponents of natural interaction, Monty Roberts and Kelly Marks, demonstrate their early work in a cage, even in this situation the horse still has a sense of personal space.

Remember, in the USA, which is the source of natural horsemanship, much of the work is done outside, the horse is allowed room, restraint is not dependent on a bit, but rather on a head collar and rope The length of the restraint rope, fixed to a head collar enables the horse to play as it wishes without either the handler pulling the horse off balance, or communicating the handler's fear of being harmed, which is immediately sensed by the horse; both can occur easily if the rope is so short that handler restraint brings the horse inward, off balance. Handling a horse also requires the handler to appreciate the inherited traits with which the horse is born, all of which are present from the moment of birth.

The programmed brain

The horse, unlike man, is born neurologically programmed for survival at birth. It can stand within minutes of being born, balance, move and suckle. All prey animals are described as precocial, this means that imprinting, or the programming of the brain is immediate. At birth, the foal immediately both visualises and memorises anything that moves (in nature, its dam) and the response of the brain is to make the foal follow and respect its dam. Early imprinting, for example attitude to strange things (man), general reactions to the world it has just entered, are shaped in a very short time, within hours of birth, and are permanently retained. Thus the best time to 'join up' with the foal is within a few hours of birth.

Body language

Each species enjoys its own unique body language, that of the horse is instinctively understood by its fellows. For the human observer many of the signals are very subtle and it is only by continued observation that it is possible to learn to 'read' them.

Reactions

All prey species possess the ability for rapid reaction. This is necessary even for the survival of domesticated animals; the horse still displays the fastest reaction time of domesticated animals, which includes perception and appropriate reaction.

Flight

The natural instinct of the horse is to run away from *any stimuli* which evokes fear.

Fight

If it is unable to run the horse will resort to fighting restraint if the fear reaction is evoked.

Perception

In their natural habitat horses need to be highly perceptive. In domestication this perception is often incorrectly considered as stupidity, but this is incorrect, for the horse detects presumed danger when compared to man through increased perception via the senses, which include sight, hearing, smell, touch and taste.

Memory

Horses need to be educated in such a manner that neither pain nor fear are evoked, as both of these will trigger the horse's natural responses – fight followed by flight. The movements asked of the horse must be carefully taught for the horse does not forget.

Often it is a lack of understanding on the part of the handler during early imprinting which results in responses from the horse which we consider inappropriate. Consider the foal, handled well at birth, with fear of man overcome, which is led to the field in a head collar, and/or shown in hand. In both of these situations, the foal often out-walks the handler; restraint from head collar and lead rope, even if the latter is centrally secured, causes the animal to turn the head slightly to the left, or toward the handler. The foal is then turned away to mature.

The animal is brought up to begin early training. The tack is put on, and pressure behind the ears and above the nostrils from the cavesson, similar to that experienced when led as a foal, evokes the brain response. The animal turns the head left, this response having been imprinted when led as a foal.

Later, in order to remain upright when lunged on a circle, the animal may have to track out with the hind quarters. This pattern, used when working on a circle, will be imprinted in the movement area of the brain. Ridden on a circle, the horse will track out just as it did on the lunge *because that is what it learned to do.*

Learning

Early traumatic experiences will be retained as fear, but if early experience can be made novel and interesting, then curiousity will overcome fear and the experience will be imprinted as acceptable. This is one of the principles taught and explained by Monty Roberts.

Learning and memory complement each other and the secret of interaction is to be certain the horse appreciates that which is required, and also that exactly the same commands/requests are given to achieve a repetition of the learned activity.

Desensitising reactions

Fortunately horses do learn to ignore situations which evoked early fear, traffic for example. However, the fact that the rapid response reactions are always present should never be ignored. Consider the many reports of cases where a horse has suddenly bolted, often on the road, and the rider response is usually, 'he's never been bad in traffic'.

Equine hierarchy

The horse expects and appreciates leadership, in the natural state there is a hierarchy of dominance, often the lead mare. The domesticated animal will respond and feel secure when given directions by the handler. Should an animal consider its self the dominant subject then subtle methods to reverse this trend are required.

Movement control

In nature the horse uses movements, other than the normal gaits of walk, trot, canter and gallop, not only to avoid predators, but also to make threatening or respectful advances toward others in the herd. The movement co-ordinations are there from birth, already imprinted in the brain. As previously described, man invokes and harnesses these pre-ordained responses by the use of 'aids'.

Man is able to achieve the desired result when riding using the learned 'aids' and by educating and conditioning both the muscles which stabilise the body frame or axial skeleton, and the groups responsible for movement.

When training an untutored horse, one major stumbling block is the introduction of the circle. This is not natural to, nor is it used by, the wild horse. The co-ordination required is extremely demanding and the introduction of circling, should, in an ideal training regime, be introduced later rather than early which is so often the case.

Organisation of the body

Appreciation of the horse's mind is only the beginning of an overview of the interaction of all the body systems required in order to ensure a healthy horse. A basic knowledge of the structure of the horse will help the reader appreciate the complexity of the interaction between the various systems of the body and the ingredients which need to be assembled and assimilated to maintain the living being. It is also important to have an awareness of the problems which can occur should the normal interaction between cells or body systems cease or become ineffective.

Cells

Life requires that maintenance and internal stability of all the systems creating the whole are conserved. Cells are the basic unit of all life. They are controlled by and respond to stimuli which may be chemical, electrical and magnetic. Life begins with the meeting of sperm and ova, the resultant single, fertilised cell divides and sub-divides to form a fetus. The raw materials required for fetal growth are absorbed from the blood of the mother directed through the placenta, during pregnancy. Unwanted substances cannot pass through the walls of the placental vessels and are effectively filtered out to avoid harming the growing fetus.

It is obvious that if the mare is able to find, or is fed, the required ingredients during pregnancy, that the foal when born will be healthy and the mare's milk will contain the nutrients needed by the foal. A mare who fares badly during pregnancy will be forced to draw upon her own internal reserves, thus she becomes weak and may deliver an under-nourished foal. It must be appreciated that problems of growth and development may have had their beginnings *in utero*. The natural horse will instinctively search for what is lacking. (Why do pregnant women have cravings?) An appreciation of the fact 'that what you do not put in you will not get out' is very important to your horse.

As the original cell divides and sub-divides into trillions of new cells, differentiation takes place and cells remodel to exhibit characteristics peculiar to their eventual function. Once those cells with similar characteristics are clumped together they form a body tissue or body system.

Cells have a number of fascinating aspects:

- Each individual cell is as complex as a galaxy in space.
- Each type of body tissue exhibits a particular cell clumping or pattern; some tissues are composed of several cell types, others of a single cell type.
- Cells reproduce.
- Some types of cell are continuously on the move within their environment. Blood cells move around the body mass within the circulatory system, others cell types migrate in response to stimuli, moving via the medium of the fluid present between all cell masses, known as extra-cellular fluid.
- Cells manufacture.
- Cells recycle.
- Cells secrete and excrete.
- Cells can destroy.
- Cells can repair damage.

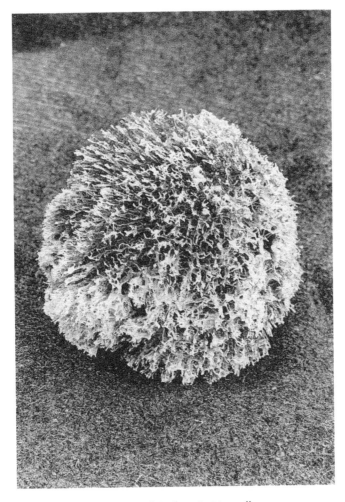

Fig. 2.2 A sponge is composed of a group of similar primitive cells.

- Each cell type has a predetermined lifespan; as they die they are replaced, within the healthy organism, by an exact replica.

To illustrate a cell is almost impossible. Photographs make them appear flat! Far from it, cells are designed in many shapes (see Fig. 2.2). The cells which form bone resemble a honeycomb, others can be round, oblong, square, some have a single tail, others many tails or projections.

Skeleton

The skeleton (see Fig. 2.3) creates the underlying frame around and in which the body mass is built; the bones of the frame are joined in a manner that achieves stability but allows movement. The frame also functions to encase and protect vital organs and to provide a platform for soft tissue attachment.

Bone is a dense connective tissue, its structure impregnated with bone salts (chiefly calcium carbonate and calcium phosphate); these give a certain rigidity but bone retains a flexibility without which it would break down under stress. Mineral salts are stored in bone where the outer shell, built in layers arranged in a concentric manner, is called

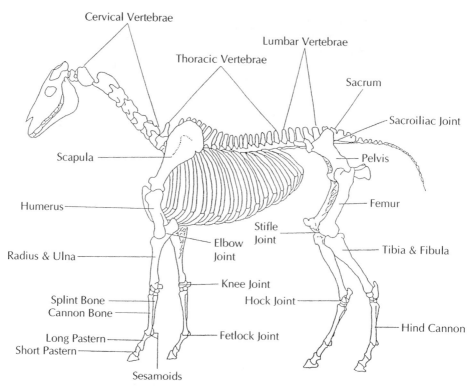

Fig. 2.3 Diagram of a horse skeleton.

compact bone. Beneath the compact bone is a network or mesh arrangement somewhat similar to a honey comb named the marrow; marrow, a site for the manufacture of cells, fills the central or *medullary cavity* in all long bones. These bone factories are very important as bone marrow manufactures erythrocytes, the red oxygen-transporting cells. Without oxygen, cell function is impossible.

All bones are encased by an outer connective tissue layer the *periosteum*. This tough membrane is used by ligaments, tendons and muscles as a means of anchorage. It also supports the vessels required to feed and nourish the bone; for bone, just like all other tissue, is constantly rebuilding, feeding and cleansing. To achieve this a plexus of blood vessels is ingeniously incorporated around and within the structure; with a main artery entering each bone via a canal called the *nutrient foramen.*

Joints

Joints are the point at which a bone surface designed to allow movement meets the similar surface of an adjoining bone or number of bones. The opposing surfaces are covered with a tissue called *hyaline* or *articular cartilage*. This semi-opaque, self-lubricating surface is constructed in a manner which allows it to withstand considerable pressure.

Joints are enclosed within an outer envelope or capsule and the hollow space created is filled with a lubricant liquid called *synovial fluid* (joint oil). The encapsulating membrane supports an inner layer of cells which manufacture and secrete joint oil in partnership with the hyaline covering of the opposing bone ends.

Unfortunately, one of the causes of lameness is the irreparable breakdown of the hyaline cartilage, often in the distal limb joints and particularly in the fetlock (ankle) joints.

The hyaline cartilage found in the joints of the horse appears inadequate to withstand the levels of joint compaction generated by the demands of modern competition.

The design of individual joints differs, some are described as hinge, these enable movement in two directions only, while the ball-and-socket design allows multi-directional movement.

Joint flexibility

It is important always to remember that the horse is a naturally developed running species which has adapted over millions of years to ensure speed for survival, while changing from a four-, to a three- and finally to a one-toed animal. The distal limb joints (knee to ground, hock to ground) are dependent on flexibility for economic function, this flexibility being governed by tendon extensibility. The front legs of the horse equate to the middle finger of the human hand, the back legs to the middle toe of the human foot. As support of these areas is achieved by tendons, ligaments and balance, it makes sense to keep the load these digits bear to a minimum. Another feature of the horse which is sometimes not appreciated is the fact that the bones of joints do not lock into one another, as the pieces of a jigsaw, but rather are suspended by their soft tissue structures – muscle, tendons and ligaments – which can be imagined as beautifully developed springs. Inadequate preparation of these soft tissue structures leads to damaging compressive factors within joints, which may manifest as irreversible changes, particularly as the hyaline cartilage coating the articular surfaces of all joints is extremely thin in the equine. The hyaline cartilage did not develop, nor was designed to, in order to accommodate to the continuous weight bearing and concussive forces experienced by the new-age horse, for in the natural horse, concussion from speed occurred for much shorter time periods.

Ligaments

Ligaments span joints. They are flexible but not elastic as their role is to add strength and support to joints both internally (for example, the *ligamentum teres* of the hip and the *cruciate ligaments* of the stifle) and externally, where they limit the movement range of a joint to that required and which the shape of the opposing bone ends can comfortably sustain. A final role of ligaments, not yet entirely understood, is to assist in joint movement by loading with kinematic energy on stretch, then discharging the energy during motion and thereby assisting a joint to return to its normal resting position.

Ligaments that are damaged are described as *sprained*. The damage is usually the result of severe overstretching. It is almost impossible to correct such a situation as, unfortunately, ligaments, unlike most other connective tissues, do not remodel to their original form.

Muscles and tendons

Smooth muscle is found in the walls of blood vessels, the gut, the stomach and other internal organs.

Cardiac muscle is specific to the heart.

Neither of these muscle types can be controlled voluntarily, both are under the command of the autonomic nervous system.

Skeletal muscles are the muscles which ensure that the bone frame is held together. They move the body and maintain the required posture against the forces of gravity. Skeletal muscles are dependent for effective function upon a nerve supply to command their actions. In order to achieve movement the muscles must pass over one or more joints and are attached via the periosteum to bone above (origin) and below (insertion) the joint or joints they are designed to influence.

In certain body areas the muscles also use *fascia* for anchorage.

Exercise influences skeletal muscle activity, ensuring that muscles develop enabling them to perform tasks as required. For muscle to increase its capability takes time, because not only must the muscle recruit more of its contractile units but those units need an efficient supply of fuel and also require waste removal. In order for this to occur tiny blood vessels called capillaries must proliferate through the building muscle.

In the limbs, muscles originating above the knees and hocks of the horse modify their structure as they near these joints, their fibres becoming increasingly strong and compact, in such a way that the tissue eventually resembles a hawser. This structure is named a *tendon*. Equine limb tendons examined microscopically demonstrate a crimp-like formation allowing for stretch and recoil when subjected to the intense demands created as the angle of pastern to ground at gallop is forced from approximately 45° to an angle of 90° (see Fig. 2.4).

The tendons of the lower or distal limbs have no mechanism to maintain an ambient central or core temperature. The heat within their core is generated by work at fast paces when the structure is being subjected to continual stretch and recoil and rapidly reaches a critical level. Any structure becomes fragile at high temperature, thus an excessive rise in the core temperature of the working tendon is considered to be one of the many reasons that may contribute to tendon breakdown.

Until recently it was considered that damaged tendons, whatever the reason for the tissue destruction, could never regain their original characteristics following injury. However, experimentation with the injection of stem cells into damaged tendon tissue is demonstrating improved natural repair.

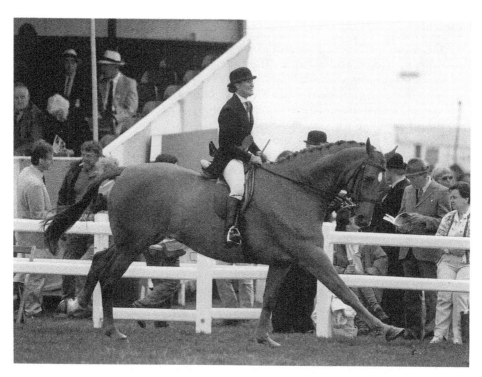

Fig. 2.4 The pastern of the near fore lies nearly parallel to the ground with the sesamoid bones momentarily taking full body weight. The tendons of that limb are at full stretch.

The cardiovascular system (heart and blood vessels)

Haemoglobin and red blood cells

In any training programme the regular monitoring of the profile of cell populations, derived from a blood sample, is essential. The blood can be likened to a barometer giving definite pointers to the current state of health. Of the many pointers available from a blood analysis is the level of haemoglobin.

Haemoglobin is a protein in the blood which specialises in the transportation of oxygen around the body. It is present in every red blood cell, comprising 33% of each red blood cell. The haemoglobin is able to attract oxygen molecules following their delivery to the lungs in inhaled air, and collect carbon dioxide molecular waste, for eventual excretion primarily in exhaled air.

The average thousand pound horse has in its system approximately 510 trillion blood cells circulating at any one time and you may be forgiven for beginning to wonder how you can ever train this animal to perfection. Unlike some other cell types, red blood cells do not reproduce themselves but are actually produced from a complex series of interactions in the marrow of the long bones, also in the liver and in the spleen.

The spleen

The spleen is very important to the exercising horse and can be compared to a large sponge full of blood cells. It serves as a container for healthy red blood cells and acts as a recycling yard for those blood cells which have finished their lifecycle. Just as the kidneys are able to recycle certain components and return them for reuse, so specialist capillaries in the spleen are able to break down used and dying blood cells. In an impressive display of efficiency, iron is taken from the decaying cells and transported back to the bone marrow and to the liver for reuse, passing into new cells as they are manufactured.

Under strenuous or maximal exercise conditions, a horse is often described as having got its 'second wind'. The 'second wind' occurs as a result of a contraction of the spleen, which releases a huge number of red cells into the circulating blood. The presence of these red blood cells results in immediately improved oxygen delivery, the contraction of the spleen is a reflex response to body demand.

Efficiency of the cardiovascular system

The efficiency of the red cells for oxygen delivery and carbon dioxide removal, as well as the number of these cells present in the blood, are critical to equine performance. Interval training generates vital signals to enhance the production of red cells. As the horse becomes fatigued and a state of oxygen debt occurs, demand for oxygen rises. Specialist systems recognise the necessity for more cells. The only way to ensure the arrival of extra red blood cells to the oxygen-depleted tissues is to increase the number of cells available both to carry the oxygen required for muscle activity and remove the carbon dioxide created. It is only by increasing the work demand, to initiate a natural response within the body, that this increased cell production occurs. It cannot be achieved by pumping in varied tonics or other substances said to 'improve' the production of the red cells. It is, however, certainly true that extra components may be necessary in cases of dietary deficiency or metabolic upset, in which case these components are normally given by injection and may include extra protein, iron, copper and cobalt, all of which are among the raw materials required for the manufacture of red blood cells.

A normal, well-balanced dietary intake should contain all the necessary components in adequate amounts and this is what the term a *balanced diet* means. The food, however it is supplied, nuts, mixes or cubes, should contain everything required to build the cells of all the tissues and to supply 'fuel'.

As the condition of your horse improves you will notice a change in the haemoglobin levels. This is because the bone marrow, liver and spleen have stepped up production in response to demand. A horse which is getting less exercise demands less oxygen – lack of demand reduces the number of red cells in production.

Circulation

Blood circulates within the blood vessels throughout the body, the vessels infiltrating every single system and structure. The circulatory system can be likened to a conveyor belt as it transports cells, oxygen, fuel, protective agents, repair kits and debris, in fact every component the body needs to sustain life, around the body to cleanse, to repair and to protect itself.

The arterial system operates under high pressure which is achieved by the pumping action of the heart. Arterial blood is therefore able to act as an efficient delivery service. The blood in the veins is loaded with waste and debris; this system is under much less pressure than arterial blood and is, in part, dependent for continual flow upon inter-rupted pressures created by muscle activity. This waste is carried to various disposal units where it is processed, with usable elements being recycled and the rest excreted in the form of urine, faeces, sweat and expelled gas; the latter exiting from the lungs via the route through which air is inhaled, the trachea and nasal passages. Once the waste has been dumped, the venous blood returns to the heart, and from there to the lungs to collect oxygen, before being redirected via the arterial system for general reloading.

The delivery of 'goods' and the collection of waste occurs through the walls of the tiny blood vessels called *capillaries*. The walls of the capillaries are specially designed to allow the easy interchange of components, both to and from the various tissues and organs.

Blood is part liquid, part cellular, with the cells suspended in a liquid called *plasma*. There are different types of cells, and each family has a particular function.

- *Leucocytes* or white blood cells have several sub-divisions, each type performing a specific, pre-determined role in the defence and repair mechanisms.
- *Erythrocytes* are the red, oxygen-carrying cells.
- *Platelets* are concerned with clotting.

Damage to the wall of a blood vessel may allow blood to escape from the normally 'closed circuit' system; any blood loss which reduces the total volume is a potential dis-aster for the horse. In such an emergency the platelets activate and initiate, within the damaged area, chemical processes which convert liquid blood to a solid state, thus preventing further blood loss and closing the breach in the vessel wall.

Blood tests

Blood has been called a *body barometer*. In the laboratory, tests have established a set of normal reference values for all the various cells and substances found in blood. Blood for testing should be taken with the horse at rest (even minimal excitement changes the cell balance).

Variations from the accepted normal are studied to aid diagnosis if a problem has occurred. The values can also be used as an indicator of the general health of a horse in the absence of problems.

Laboratory tests are used to build a 'blood picture'. Knowledge of the changes in blood chemistry and the behaviour of its components is the subject of increased research. Blood taken pre- and post-exercise allows values, other than just cellular values, to be scrutinised, and it is suggested that this analysis will also assist in the

Table 2.1 Generally accepted normal reference values of equine blood.

	Thoroughbred	Non-Thoroughbred
Red blood cells (RBC) $\times 10^{12}$/1	7.0 to 13.0	5.5 to 9.5
Haemoglobin Hb/dl	10 to 18	8 to 14
White blood cells (WBC) $\times 10^9$/1	6 to 12	6 to 12
Platelets $\times 10^9$/1	200 to 400	200 to 400
Neutrophils $\times 10^9$/1		2.5 to 7.0
Lymphocytes $\times 10^9$/1		1.6 to 5.4
Monocytes $\times 10^9$/1		0.6 to 0.7

assessment of other factors – tolerance to exercise, fitness level, and recovery after competition, being just a few examples.

Only vets are allowed to take blood from a horse. Laboratory technicians then prepare and test the blood. The vet then reads the test results and is able to report on the findings. A great number of tests are possible and while you (the owner) will be given a copy of the 'blood picture', the rows of names, abbreviations and figures will mean very little unless you have been trained to interpret the findings. For example, what do the abbreviations RBC and WBC mean?

RBC = red blood cells;
WBC = white blood cells.

However, there are different types of white cells, all of which have their own accepted normal levels, and any deviation from the accepted 'normal' value is significant and to an expert is a vital piece in the jigsaw puzzle of diagnosis.

Table 2.1 gives a guide to the generally accepted 'normal' reference values of equine blood. It is not a full list of the possible biochemical estimations.

Total proteins, albumin and globulin levels can all be assessed, as can plasma, fibrogen, urea, creatinine, and enzymes, one of which, *creatinine kinase* (CPK), is associated with, among other conditions, muscle damage.

Blood values differ both within individuals and within breeds. It is the job of skilled personnel to analyse and report on the factual evidence supplied from the tested blood samples, as body conditions can be recognised by collating the variance from the accepted normal 'picture'. The 'blood picture' can also demonstrate if there has been a muscle breakdown in response either to exercise or trauma, whether an infection is present or if the animal is recovering from infection. A wide range of vital information can be obtained from a blood sample.

Another reason for monitoring blood profiles, is that certain tissues which are under stress but which have not yet broken down, release chemicals. Analysis of these chemicals by an expert is another diagnostic aid.

The reading of the blood and reporting on the health picture is the job of a highly qualified technician. Money used to pay for blood tests is never wasted. Tests should be taken at regular intervals and discussed with your veterinarian throughout any training programme.

Lymphatic system

The body is composed largely of fluid which needs constantly to be moving or circulating. Lymph is a fluid similar to blood plasma and contains proteins and other substances all of which are needed by body components. The vessels of the lymphatic system associate very closely with all veins, the maze of lymphatic vessels lying alongside the plexus of veins. 'Filtering stations', or clumps of *lymph nodes* are strategically sited within the network of lymphatic vessels. These lymph nodes help combat infection and disease by filtering toxins and manufacturing scavenging cells. If excessively activated by the presence of irritants they swell, with those sited superficially becoming visually obvious and often painful when palpated.

All fluids within tissue, not collected by the veins, diffuse into the lymphatic vessels, and migrate slowly to a vessel called the *thoracic duct*. From there, via veins called the *innominate veins*, the fluids are returned to the main stream circulation.

The lymphatic system has no pressure pump to assist fluid movement; flow is partly dependent on the variation of pressures occurring within the muscle tissues created by movement. As the equine distal limbs are devoid of muscle fluids tend to pool causing excessive swelling.

Until recently, there has been little research on lymphatic flow in the horse. A recent publication resulting from work in Germany by Dirk Berens von Rautenfeld describes the system in detail and suggests therapeutic methods (see General Bibliography, page 231).

Respiration

Respiration is often only considered from the viewpoint of oxygen uptake within the lungs, but the term respiration more accurately refers to the interchange of gases throughout the body, at cellular level. The term includes carbon dioxide, a gas which, beside being present in inhaled air, is a waste produced during cellular respiration.

Oxygen is an essential ingredient for all body processes. In muscle tissue, oxygen combines chemically with body fuels, in particular with glucose, to provide the energy required for muscle activity.

Oxygen is absorbed into the blood within the lungs, taken from the air drawn in through the upper respiratory tract. This tract consists of the nasal passages, the larynx, the pharynx and the trachea, which, on entering the thoracic cage, sub-divides into two major bronchi, one for each lung. The bronchi divide and sub-divide, becoming smaller and smaller, until, as terminal bronchioles, they redesign to become the air sacs or *alveoli*. The specialist walls of the alveoli allow the diffusion of gases both into and from tiny blood vessels, the capillaries, which enmesh their walls. Thus, through the walls of both alveoli and capillaries, oxygen passes into the circulatory system and similarly carbon dioxide is expelled from the circulatory system through them. Both gases are transported in the blood stream by the red cells or erythrocytes.

Lack of oxygen and reduced carbon dioxide removal will reduce the horse's performance dramatically. Reduced oxygen delivery can be traced to many factors: for example upper airway disease, or the inability of the thoracic cage, within which the lungs are installed, to expand. Diet must also be considered. Is the horse receiving the iron necessary for haemoglobin synthesis? Depletion in the body of this mineral which is essential for red cell function, results in poor transportation by the blood cells of both oxygen and carbon dioxide. Within the lung tissue, irritant particles of dust can cause damage to the fragile walls of the air sacs. Such damage will stop gas molecules passing through those walls for collection prior to transportation and conversely there will be reduced carbon dioxide removal. It follows in situations involving inefficient oxygen uptake, transportation to the body tissues by red blood cells waiting in the capillary vessels is reduced, carbon dioxide waste builds up and a train of unhelpful chemical reactions can result.

The respiratory and cardiovascular systems are inextricably linked to service the body's requirement for oxygen. To attempt to ensure an adequate oxygen supply, in-built safety mechanisms control the rate and depth of respiration, as well as the rate at which the heart beats in order to propel blood through the arterial system. However, these safety mechanisms are useless if the flow of air from the exterior is reduced, curtailed or polluted.

Tissue fatigue occurs early in the absence of oxygen and inefficient carbon dioxide removal.

Expelling warmed air during expiration also assists in maintaining body temperature. The misting fans used at venues where horses are competing in conditions of excessive temperature, ensure that inhaled air is cool, reducing the temperature of the blood as it circulates through the lung tissues, and moist, to help reduce dehydration secondary to fluid loss, as the horse attempts to cool itself by sweating.

The nervous system

The components of the nervous system control all body functions – communication, recording, analysis and action following analysis, control of all systems, control of movement, control of the heart, response to pain and stimuli, control of temperature and so on, the list is infinite.

The nervous system is the first to be developed in the growing fetus. At birth, the foal arrives with several, existing co-ordinated actions programmed in the brain; it can stand, balance in standing, suck, and recognise its mother; it can also smell, and run with the herd if required; then, from the moment of birth, incredibly rapid learning processes take place. Repeated actions are logged in the brain, the messages invoked by the actions having been passed by nerves in the tissues to the spinal cord and thence to the brain.

As previously stated *logged actions become accepted as normal, thus if a foal is always led with its head turned toward the handler, the brain will accept and register this as the norm, i.e. a position to be adopted whenever the horse wears a halter or later a bridle.*

Central nervous system

The central nervous system consists of the brain and spinal cord. For maximum protection these are housed within cavities surrounded by bone – the brain within the skull and the spinal cord within the vertebral column. Both brain and spinal cord are wrapped in three layers of protective tissue and are suspended in fluid. Specialist *cranial nerves* arise directly from the brain and leave the skull, each via its own aperture. In the horse there are twelve pairs of these nerves which control highly specialised functions such as smell, sight and hearing. Destruction of, compression to, disease within, or any disturbance of the normal function of central nervous tissue is irreversible and is extremely serious for the horse.

The autonomic nervous system

This section of the nervous system can be described as an automatic system – it is crucial to life. Communication with appropriate centres in the brain is constant, but, unlike the peripheral nervous system, not all the branches of the system arise from the spinal cord. The continual stream of commands and messages ensures that the body remains viable with out any voluntary effort or consideration on the part of animal or human. The system controls all the basic functions of life, respiration, metabolism, digestion, the cardiovascular system and thermal regulation to name but a few. The sensors of this system are located throughout the entire body mass, many sited in the connective tissue, known as *fascia* which both enmeshes and envelopes every system in a continuous, unbroken sheet.

Exponents of acupressure and acupuncture consider that the autonomic system responds to acu stimulation and it is suggested that the relative positions of acu and trigger points are similar. It is hypothesised that the autonomic system is also stimulated by the massage technique skin rolling (see page 94) due to the direct effects on the subcutaneous fascia. This technique has been renamed/reinvented many times but the principle behind it has remained similar.

Peripheral nervous system

At the intersections between each of the individual bones forming the vertebral column, a pair of *spinal nerves* branch off, one to the left side of the body one to the right. The nerves originate from the spinal cord housed within the canal formed by the vertebrae. These nerves are in continual communication with the spinal cord and, via this structure, with the brain. The nerves pass outward into the body mass, elongating and sub-dividing as they go, eventually enmeshing the entire structure within an elaborate control network.

Pressure or disturbance to nervous tissue lying within the body mass outside the central complex of brain or spinal cord effectively reduces and even cuts communication to and from all the structures serviced by the nerve or nerves involved; muscle tissue is unable to function in the absence of signals from its *motor nerve*.

In these circumstances where the nervous tissue is damaged or compromised, normally recorded sensations such as heat, cold, pain or position in space are not appreciated; the circulation within the affected area is impaired and the skin area supplied by the nerve involved cannot react normally to external stimuli.

The nervous system is distributed in a known pattern with the skin surface divided into segments known as *dermatomes*; reduced sensation within a dermatome enables identification of the compromised nerve. For those offering therapy to horses, knowledge of the muscles supplied by the identified nerve should enable the installation of an appropriate exercise regime to target and thereby rebuild the muscles involved.

Digestive system

The digestive system refines and processes all the substances the horse eats. Just like any 'factory', the body needs raw ingredients to sustain production. A factory usually has the required raw materials delivered ready prepared for immediate use, but this is not the case in the horse which needs to process its food, and chewing is the first stage of this refining process. Chewing is also essential in activating the digestive processes. Pulverising plant matter in the mouth uses energy, as does the refining and selection of the all components within the food that the horse needs: the nutrients, proteins, carbohydrates, fats, minerals, vitamins and water. Energy is wasted if a diet is badly balanced. If it is too dry it is hard for the horse to break it down, or if it has insufficient bulk. Energy is also wasted if the horse is unable to chew correctly because of tooth problems. Digestion within the stomach and intestine is aided by saliva and secretions manufactured in other organs. These organs are also able to store nutrients for future use. The digestive process which started in the mouth continues through the intestines, with extraction of useful ingredients, until the waste is compacted and expelled as droppings.

The digestive organs, or intestines, are formed as a tube. The long and convoluted structure is contiguous with the body's outer surface, through the lips and lining of the mouth at its beginning to the anus at the end of the digestive system, the tube leads from the mouth into the body cavity. For descriptive purposes, the tube is divided into named sections: oesophagus, stomach, duodenum, small intestine, jejunum, caecum, ileum, colon, small colon, then the rectum ending at the anus. This, the final valve in the system, is sited between the tube and exterior, with the walls of the anus blending, as did the lips, with the body skin. This design prevents any toxic material entering the abdominal cavity should something poisonous be eaten or inadvertently created.

Dimensions of the tube within the body vary depending on both its particular function and position within the digestive system. The tube (intestines) moves continuously in a wave-like ripple, moving its contents in a continuous unidirectional flow from stomach to anus. For safety, as previously stated, the tube does not open into the body cavity, and as such it is not truly part of the internal architecture of the body in the same way, for example, as the liver, spleen or kidneys.

The kidneys and bladder

The kidneys are not merely organs of excretion, they are essential for the maintenance of the correct acid–base balance of the blood and tissue fluids. They also function to conserve metabolic products being excreted as waste, with the ability to convert these components, taken from the liquid they filter, back into usable assets.

After filtration within the kidneys, unessential chemicals suspended in liquid known as urine, pass down the urethra to the bladder, from where, when sufficient is collected, in response to commands from the autonomic nervous system, the urine is voided to the exterior. The colour, texture and smell of the urine are important, in a healthy horse the liquid should be clear and odourless.

As with blood, urine can be examined, and there are a set of base values for the components and variations from normal which may indicate health problems; the presence of stimulants or any type of prohibited compounds is also detectable.

Summary

This text has provided a brief description of the body systems of the horse. To summarise:

- the frame is bone;
- muscles move the frame as commanded by the nervous system;
- the digestive system extracts the required nutrients from the food;
- the circulatory and respiratory systems deliver and excrete;
- the nervous system controls and commands the balanced interlinking of the functions of all the systems which deal with delivery, disposal, feeding, building, defending, seeing, smelling, responding, keeping warm, resting, moving, excreting and breathing, in fact every body function.

It is important to reflect on the fact that the body functions as a whole, and those who try to influence its systematic activities for their personal pleasure and enjoyment must try to comprehend this.

Everything, from the smallest cell to the largest organ creating the being we call a horse, its response to its human master as well as every feature of its make-up, is inextricably interconnected and the horse can only function to become a companion if all the complex systems not only work but if their functions and peculiarities are understood, appreciated and maintained in a healthy condition; and in order to achieve this, all the necessary ingredients must be made freely available to the horse in the correct, balanced proportions.

3 Reading Your Horse

Health pointers

It is impossible to train a horse that is not well; the animal cannot describe if it feels well or ill, it is therefore essential to learn to 'read' each animal. There are many health pointers to look out for, all of which need daily consideration, for the onset of an illness often occurs as in man for no obvious reason, the horse may be well one day and ill the next.

Stockmen always 'read' their stock and it is only possible to learn how to do this by constant observation – books can tell you what to look for, but the art of husbandry is a continuous learning curve. Look and observe day in day out until the observations become habit and it is possible to recognise and record changes without thinking, noting the condition of coat, mane and tail, eye brightness, gum colour, hoof growth, the smell, colour and amount of urine produced, the colour and texture of the droppings (faeces).

Fifty years ago, no doctor ever examined a patient without looking at their nails (hoofs), hair (mane and tail), eye, both for brightness and the colour of the lower lid, questions regarding urine and faeces (droppings) were also routine. The value of this process is still the same, you need to learn to read the condition of your horse through constant observation.

Mechanical objects are continually updated, consider the leap from early computers to the situation today where we enjoy instant communication through broadband. Most people live in an instant-fix, throw-away society, rather than a society where one is required through necessity to save, conserve, recycle in order to survive. Today, we are also subjected to continual pressures through advertisement and common sense seems to have reduced, with many people believing unrealistic claims for enhanced performance as a result of product or method 'X'. There are in reality no training aids, special rugs, specialised gadgets, coat shines, special diets, bandages or therapies which will accelerate a naturally ordained order of progression, developed over millions of years, in order to produce an equine athlete.

Horses are not machines with replaceable components, they are a miracle of chemical interactions and biomechanical engineering. There is no instant fix in the preparation of the horse as a ridden athlete.

The horse is designed for speed, generally in order to avoid predators, when living, as intended in the evolutionary sense, in the wild. In a natural state, with no specialist training, the horse is capable of performing at above the speed of a trained human, running at around 45 mph (70 km/h), and is able to maintain that speed over a considerable distance. The zebra, first cousin to the horse, is known to run for up to a hundred miles after scenting distant water when local rains have failed.

To achieve movement, particularly speed, the frame must be light but stable, and muscle activity in the limbs, whose function is to move the body mass, must be economical.

In order to achieve this, the tissues rely on stretch and recoil, performing rather like lengths of high quality elastic. This stretch and recoil is only efficient if the bone frame, or axial skeleton is stable.

Prior to introducing the domesticated horse to any training programme, be it that suggested by Monty Roberts, or the increasing number of emerging natural horsemen, the ability to read the horse is required. To learn to read a horse takes time, and those skilled are described as having an 'eye for a horse'. To develop this skill necessitates honing the powers of observation.

Monty Roberts has 'an eye for a horse', but how did this develop? First, he lived with groups of horses on the rodeo circuit, he watched their behaviour. Disliking many of the training and horsemanship methods he saw, he tried other methods which were unconventional, logging everything – response, mood, reaction, pain evidence; then, when dismissed as a crank, he went to live with a group of wild horses to expand his knowledge through observation of the behavioural traits of the horse living in its natural state.

To become a true horseman requires consideration of the following in the horse:

- general health;
- diet;
- skeletal preparation;
- muscle preparation;
- joint flexibility;
- balance;
- adequate exposure to unfamiliar situations.

General health

As previously stated, it is impossible to work successfully with a horse that is not well. The horse has no verbal means to indicate its current state of health. The animal may be irritable because it slept badly, has muscle ache following the previous day's work, or, in the mare, has pre-menstrual tension (yes, they have this!).

The art of husbandry is a continuous learning curve. Decide your own routine, follow *your chosen* observation pattern, use it every time you look at your horse until your daily reading (observation) becomes automatic.

Learn to note the condition of coat, mane, tail, brightness of eye, hoof growth, gum colour, smell, colour and volume of urine produced, smell, colour and texture of droppings. Traditional Chinese medicine examines the whole patient.

Important observations in both the human and animal are:

Human	Horse	Possible cause of problem
nails	hooves	mineral lack
hair	mane and tail	poor health/diet
tongue/gums	black gums or stained teeth	mineral lack
skin	dry coat and tight skin texture	dehydration

Questions are asked about stools (droppings) and urine.

Worming

Before starting on a training programme it is sensible to treat your animal for worms. Current indications are that many horses are becoming resistant to the conventional de-worming programmes; the offices of all veterinary practitioners will provide up-to-date information on the subject, either by leaflet or conversation (see diatomaceous earth, worm effects, page 33).

Injections

It is also sensible to make certain that a horse is up to date with all the necessary injections before starting work. Many horses feel 'off colour' for several days after their 'flu jabs, some may develop mild coughs, even a runny nose. They must be given time to recover fully, for at least two to three days before going back into or starting work.

(While riders rarely require treatment for worms unless they have visited areas of the world in which human worms are common, far too many grooms and riders neglect their own immunity injections, it is *essential* to ensure that *tetanus protection* is regularly updated.)

Feet

Hoof growth, texture and appearance is, just as for the human nail, a major health indicator. 'No foot, no horse', is such a true statement; the condition of the hoof is critical for optimum performance.

The hoof is the first part of the body to make contact with the ground at all gaits. It is the weight-bearing base of each limb, its shape determines the angularity to the ground of the joints between the long and short pastern bones, the short pastern and the coffin bone, described in anatomy books as P1, P2, P3.

The angle of the foot to the ground obviously affects the stress angles of the bones and joints of individual limbs. Incorrect balance within an individual foot, between pairs, or even diagonal pairs of feet, changes the relationship of the affected limb/s to the body mass. This affects both balance and thrust and can be a major cause of poor performance, because the axial skeleton is forced to adjust. *However*, before starting an argument with your farrier, or if you are a bare-foot enthusiast, and want to try trimming to balance the feet of your horse to a 45° angle with even heel length, make absolutely certain the foot shape you are about to alter did not occur due to a limb imbalance. *The uneven growth may be a required response to offset a conformation fault.*

The *bulbs* of the heels are loaded with nerve sensors which continuously record information and communicate with the brain. Foot fall, limb sequence, muscle co-ordination, gravitational balance and adjustment to uneven terrain, all of these and many more physical functions require sensory (proprioceptive) input. Information concerning uneven terrain, ground condition, balance and limb co-ordination are just a few of the requirements necessitating information from the feet.

The *frog* is a pressure pump which through contraction and expansion, aids the return of venous blood from the foot and distal limb. It is designed to be in contact with the ground, to be moist and flexible, not dry and hard. Contracted heels, between which the frog lies, limit frog function. A dry frog or a diseased frog, susceptible as it is to fungal invasion such as thrush, cannot work efficiently and the entire body suffers as a result.

The *sole* of the foot should be slightly moist, as it too moves during ground impaction. The hoof is not a totally rigid structure, it deforms and reshapes to aid the dissipation and absorption of all impaction forces. As with all other body tissues the foot has its own nutritional requirements which cannot be obtained by rubbing in preparations. If the necessary components are missing because the diet is imbalanced, then the hoof will be dry, break easily and grow slowly in the same way human nails behave if there is a nutritional deficiency or following illness.

Trimming feet

Extending periods between trimming feet is a false economy. You should never try to save money by elongating the periods between either shoeing or regular trimming, even horses turned away in the field, barefooted for their holiday, must have regular foot attention. A horse with poor quality feet will always have problems. It will only ever be a poor quality athlete and poor quality feet also result in secondary joint problems as the horse endeavours to reduce the discomfort in its feet, often doing so by landing incorrectly at the expense of the limb joints, particularly the fetlock joints (ankles).

Read the feet. The outer hoof wall should be smooth and slightly oily to the touch.

The hoof wall may exhibit individual, ring-like bulges, running around the outer surface of the wall from heel to heel. These indicate growth of the foot at a time of change in the horse's nutrition. If the texture of the growth on the wall above the individual rings is smooth with an oily texture this indicates an improved diet containing hoof nutrients, or if the growth appears dry, possibly rough, this indicates that the horse's diet lacked ingredients. These rings are sometimes called laminitic rings, although their presence does not indicate that laminitis in the true disease form is present.

Seek professional advice before rushing in to dietary supplementation if you observe hoof wall changes. Balancing nutrition is not a 'hit and miss' affair. The laminitis and hoof health centre near Wootton Bassett in Wiltshire runs a help line. Robert Eustace, the director of the centre is both a vet and a farrier (see Useful Addresses section, page 234).

The wild horse wears the hoof continually. Most of them, if the Mustang and Exmoor ponies are taken as examples, retain a near perfect foot, partly because their diet ensures growth, but not overgrowth and the varied terrain over which they move will ensure that the horse moves on areas with surfaces of an abrasive quality.

It is important to repeat that the shape of foot may be determined by structural deformities within the limb and this may be the cause of the apparent imbalance in the foot.

Incorrect balance which has not developed to compensate for structural deformities can lead to secondary joint problems, as the animal in question endeavours to avoid sub-clinical discomfort by landing incorrectly at the expense of other limb joints.

Problems with the feet

A *boxy* foot usually occurs if the horse has for some reason reduced weight through that foot when standing.

A *flat* foot may indicate the foot takes most weight when standing.

These variations are most common in front feet, the horse often having a flat foot on one side, and a boxy foot on the other.

Squared-off toes are common in hind feet. One foot or both may be affected. The horse may be lazy, slopping along, making no effort to lift its hind feet; there may be sub-clinical pain in a limb joint of the affected hind leg, often the hock; or a habit pattern, secondary to a past discomfort, often in the hindquarter musculature, has been established.

Under-run heels, an over-long toe forces weight backwards onto the heels, over time structural deformities occur, changing the angle of foot to ground. This is detrimental to the entire limb, changing joint angles and increasing tendon stresses. Try pointing your toes upward taking all the weight on your heels, walk first, then try to run with your foot in this position, you will feel strain and discomfort in all of your limb components.

Long toes and under-run heels in a horse cause more problems in joints, tendons and ligaments than almost any other condition.

Increased growth of a medial or lateral heel may occur if the knee is offset.

The *angle* of hoof wall from coronet to ground may indicate uneven weight bearing. A very straight wall can indicate that the other side of the foot is taking more weight indicated by a lateral flare.

Feet may be flared out on one side. This is usually associated with unbalanced ground contact and incorrect break over. Sometimes secondary to a corn, other causes may be conformational, due to imbalance of the foot, sub-clinical pain in the foot or limb, *habit*, the latter often associated with a problem which has resolved. *Always remember: the horse rapidly adopts incorrect movement patterns if avoiding pain and retains those patterns until taught to re-establish the pre-pain patterns of movement.*

Barefoot

Barefoot, rather than shod, is becoming an increasingly popular choice for horse owners. The natural horse is barefoot but, remember, it can choose both its route and pace over ground.

If your horse has previously been shod and you decide to leave it barefoot, you may well find you have a foot-sore horse for several months, while the soles and walls grow thicker as they readapt in response to new signals from the ground and a differing balance perception.

With the increasing danger of road traffic, road work is often avoided, with many horses only being ridden on artificial surfaces, or, if available, over open country. So barefoot may be your choice and given time, in many horses, their feet will eventually adapt to being un-shod, *but* do not expect to remove the shoes and find that your horse will appreciate the change immediately. If you take off your shoes when on a seaside holiday can you immediately run over pebbles or shale?

Changing the shape of the foot

Always remember that the foot expert is the farrier, and before rushing in to request a change of foot shape you should consider several things including breed characteristics. For example, it is natural for the average European dressage horse or warm blood, to have quite small feet with high heels, to change this conformation has proved disastrous in most cases. Flat TB horses from the USA have rather donkey-shaped feet when compared to the 'soup plate' shape of the original British TB; American horses need to dig for security into the dirt on which they race. However, in the UK, when racing on grass, the greater the surface area covered by the foot the less the animal sinks in.

If your farrier thinks it is a good idea to reshape the feet of your horse the process will take several months, *it cannot be achieved in one session*; *all* the structures of the foot need to readjust, rearranging their internal architecture in response to change of angulation. Look at the feet of your horse, learn to read its health and way of going from its feet.

Some problems may require specialist shoes. Discuss any problems with your farrier. Remember they were the only vets until veterinary medicine became a recognised profession, and that was not until 1844 when a Royal Charter gave recognition to The Royal College of Veterinary Surgeons.

Coat

The hair comprises a part of the skin complex, the latter being the largest organ of the body. In a horse that is healthy and correctly hydrated it should be easy to 'pick up a handful of skin' on the neck, or the area of shoulder just above the elbow.

As the coat is an integral part of the largest body organ, and remembering that all body systems inter-relate, a good sheen indicates good health. If the coat looks dull, is not silky when stroked, feels dry and/or taut, these are all indications that the general health of the horse requires attention. This is usually described as 'the horse having gone off in its coat'. If the coat is 'stary', that is, not lying flat, feels rough to the touch, is dry, or, when picked up it and the underlying skin feel taut rather than elastic, any of these findings indicate that the animal may be unwell rather than cold. In a healthy horse the coat should shimmer, shine, feel like silk to the touch and have a rapid, elastic recoil.

The individual hairs of the coat work in partnership with the sweat glands, also components of the skin, and both assist in temperature regulation. Each individual hair possesses its own minute muscle; as the animal becomes cold, these muscles contract, raising the individual hairs in order to trap air between the hairs and thereby create a layer of insulation. To the human eye, the coat then looks as though it is fluffed up. Have you ever seen a Shetland pony on a cold day? A perfect example of equine insulation.

In the heat the hairs lie flat, no air is trapped between them and the sweat glands begin, if so commanded by the thermal regulating system of the body, to excrete moisture, dampening the coat and achieving heat loss through evaporation, provided the ambient humidity is not excessive. Moisture loss equals electrolyte loss, and loss of sodium in particular.

Testing for dehydration

Always test for dehydration after excessive sweating.

There are two methods used to test the horse for dehydration. The first involves pinching a small section of the skin on the neck, between the thumb and fingers, holding the fold for 30 seconds then releasing. If the pinched fold is slow to return to normal then the horse lacks fluid. An immediate return to normal suggests the hydration level is of no concern.

This test has drawbacks and a second method is to push back the lower lip and press hard with a finger or thumb on the gum, keep up the pressure for approximately 30 seconds, if the hydration levels are normal the pink tinge of the gum should restore immediately, if the area remains white the horse is dehydrated.

Coat products and greasing

Show sheen and other similar products which laminate individual hairs, interfere with natural temperature regulation. Udder cream or other preparations liberally applied to limbs and belly prior to the cross country phase at Three-Day Events do the same. The resulting insulation created from this substantially reduces the area available for heat loss when temperatures are high.

The theory behind the use of these creams appears to stem from the idea that the horse will 'slip' over the fences; get real, if you wish that to happen grease the fences! In the slippery pole competition the pole is greased not the competitor's feet.

Greasing has become accepted in the Event scene, although it was certainly not used in the early days of the sport. Common sense suggests smear with grease if you wish to insulate, after all that is the method used by cross-channel swimmers, but not if you wish to retain natural temperature control.

Mane and tail

The texture of the mane and tail vary with breed from slightly coarse to silky, but in all breeds the hair should feel pliable to touch and brush out easily.

A dry feel and/or odd reddish hairs, or reddish ends to some hairs can indicate mineral lack. This requires expert advice and/or discussion with local farmers regarding supplementation needed by their stock.

Gums

The gum colour should be pinkish, not white. Very white gums are often an indication of a low level of haemoglobin. Stained gums and teeth suggest mineral lack.

Eyes

The eyes should be bright, their expression alert. A pale interior of the lower lid and dull eyes indicate that all is not well.

Eye expression tells a lot, learn to read them for signs of pleasure, irritation, as well as health.

Urine

The urine should be clear, not overly yellow, and plentiful. Scant cloudy urine, or very dark urine requires investigation and probably attention to diet, and in particular to protein levels in feed.

A strong smell of ammonia in the horse's box also indicates that the urine is not normal since normal urine should not smell. Neither should it be scanty or cloudy and it should be passed as an easy, full flow, as though a tap is running, not dripping.

Dark urine passed after competition usually indicates a state of dehydration. The dark colour may also occur following a rapid breakdown of energy components, secondary to the fact that the animal has been asked to perform at a level too demanding for its current state of fitness.

The kidneys are a vital organ and were never ignored in husbandry in past times. A product which is no longer available, saltpetre, was, in good yards, put into the Sunday night feed to flush out the kidneys and avoid Monday morning disease (probably akin to tying up). The amount required described as enough to cover one side of a 'three penny piece'!

As in the analysis of blood there are known levels for the components found in normal urine. Analysis is a method of testing used both as a health indicator and to detect prohibited substances.

Droppings (faeces)

The quality of the droppings should be noted daily. The droppings will change colour according to diet, those of the grazing animal usually have a greenish tinge, those of the stabled animal a brownish colour.

The presence of whole food particles such as corn, oats, barley, indicate a tooth problem – primary grinding is not occurring and when this happens, digestion is affected, with nutrition becoming inadequate as the ingested food cannot be correctly broken down or absorbed. Droppings should not have an unpleasant smell, or be either too dry or too loose.

Dry droppings suggest hydration levels in the body are low. Loose, cow-pat type droppings need serious consideration for the hindgut is the area in which the main absorption of nutrients takes place, and 'hurry' of the droppings through this area reduces uptake of vital nutrients.

Ideally, the droppings should not smell and should present as well formed, moist pellets. Hard, round pellets indicate the need for increased moisture, this situation can often be addressed by damping food or hay.

A change of food, worming and young fresh grass will all affect digestion, reading both droppings and urine will indicate current digestive factors.

Summary

You know how you, as a person, feel before becoming unwell, you learn to read the indications; the horse feels much the same, but the only way that it can indicate any problems are through the medium of mood change, changes in performance ability and finally, overall body changes. *Your skill as the keeper is to learn to observe and act upon these signals.*

It is essential to learn to read your animal, it is an integral part of horsemanship and husbandry. Your responsibility to your horse is to learn the subtle signals the horse emits, and they are subtle. You must accept that like yourself a horse will change moods, feel tired, ache after new physical tasks and will not always react as you require. This ability to 'read' mood and general condition is the first and one of most important of the skills required in good horsemanship. The second skill is in understanding the necessity for a stable body frame (skeleton) and well-prepared muscles.

Appreciation of these factors will go some way to helping in your understanding of this complex animal but nothing can be achieved unless the horse is healthy, thus feeding/diet requires consideration before any form of training can be considered.

4 Diet

Only time, performance evaluation and the reading of an animal's condition will tell what best suits each particular horse; some cannot tolerate certain types of grain, others become unwell if sugar beet is added to their rations.

Unfortunately one of the major problems of today's balanced feeds is that while they must contain the protein, mineral, fibre levels printed on the label, there is no guarantee that the ingredients come from a similar source in each batch of feed.

Feeding a horse is part of *the art of husbandry*, and horses do not get fit, as a rider once suggested to me, without both food and activity. The client, in response to a question regarding the workload of her horse asked, 'Why does he need to work in order for me to compete? The information on the food package states that the food will keep him fit and keep him healthy'.

It is sensible to feed a horse at the same time each day. Studies have suggested that food arriving at regular intervals can improve a horse's performance by up to 40%.

If you do decide to make changes in the horse's feed, it is essential to do it slowly because the digestive system has become accustomed to a particular metabolic process; to change rapidly to another is a recipe for disaster.

The annual change over from old to new hay is a prime example, new hay, that is, hay less than six months old, should be introduced by mixing some new with some old, increasing the amount of 'new' gradually over a two to three week period. In 2007, the spring and summer were very wet and the quality of traditional hay and haylage differed widely from that made in 2006. As a result of these differences, a large number of horses, when changed overnight to the new products, 'tied up'.

Despite the pronouncements of the many feed experts, we are still a long way from understanding nutrition in any species. Look at the literature on human nutrition – fats in, fats out, this mineral, that mineral, more of this, less of that, the information continuously changes the most recent often in total contradiction to the information supplied by a previous bulletin.

The horse evolved in areas most suited to its needs, but despite an intensive search it has been impossible to find an analysis of the minerals present in those soils, of the plants available, or of the composition of the water at the time the horse evolved.

Species living naturally apparently manage to trace and absorb, in the correct balance (*very important*) their mineral requirements. For example, calcium and phosphorus are essential for the growth of new antlers in the deer, insufficiency of these minerals in their locality causes the deer to chew on their cast antlers in order to regain the necessary minerals.

Calcium and phosphorus are essential for numerous metabolic processes, including muscle activity. If not supplied in the diet the body borrows from bone and as a result can become osteoporotic.

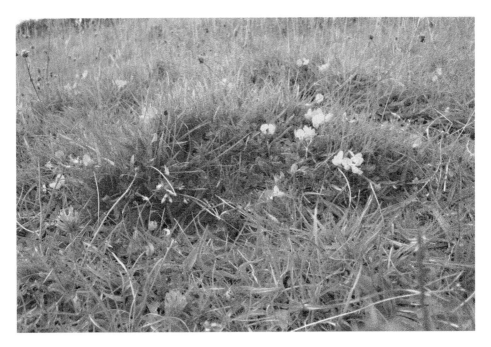

Fig. 4.1 Natural selective nutrition.

Food naturally (see Fig. 4.1)

Unlike plants, animals do not manufacture the chemicals they need, they rely directly or indirectly on plants to supply them with the necessary essentials; animal health and welfare are therefore directly dependent on plant chemistry.

When discussing feeding, the seasons of the year should be considered, for a point often overlooked is the fact that a horse is still a seasonal animal. In spring, plants emerge from their winter rest; then, drawing nutrients from the soil, begin their cycle of growth, ripening, seeding/fruiting, completing the cycle before the onset of the next winter season.

- *Spring*: a time of rich forage for all grazing animals, plants are full of nutritional elements in great concentration.
- *Summer*: this is a relaxed time, when extra condition, to see the animal through the next six months, is achieved. This extra condition is ensured due to ingestion of the ripening vegetation. The plants continue their annual cycle, drawing from the soil to manufacture the ingredients they require, then preparing to direct energy towards ensuring that their seeds will be ready to continue the cycle of existence.
- *Autumn*: by now the plants are less nutritious and becoming scarce, the horse, needing energy for everyday existence and coat growth in order to prepare for winter insulation, begins to lose summer fat.
- *Winter*: a time of scarce vegetation, the lean time, weight is lost naturally.

As nutrition is a vital part of natural horsemanship, this cycle should be taken into account. Unfortunately, many animals carry too much condition throughout the year which is detrimental to health. An Arab saying, '*the greatest enemies of the horse are rest and fat*', should be hung in every feed room!

Many horses are allowed to become far too fat and there is a misconception than an animal must be well covered, looking rather like a prize bull. Obesity in man is causing grave concern, creating as it does, many health problems. We must be sensible, for the same applies to horses. Being too fat is particularly damaging in yearlings, many of whom are undoubtedly allowed to become grossly over topped, often during their sales preparation or for the show ring, where fat seems to mean fit, and monstrous animals are shown in the ring, the extra weight they are carrying stressing every limb joint. Surely discerning judges and prospective purchasers realise how easy it is to mask conformation faults by over topping?

To save young joints and prepare them for the future, the body mass must be adequately covered but not overly so. The horse should also be provided with adequate space for movement and play at all paces. This really is very important – young animals should run out of energy and slow down by themselves rather than have to suddenly 'put on the brakes', stressing knees, hocks, stifles. Treatment is then required to control windgalls (wind puffs), where filling occurs in hocks and knees.

The feral horse of South Africa and North America grazes on mixed quality herbage; minerals are sourced from rock outcrops, the horses visiting the mineral-rich supply during their routine, seasonal migration. After two to three days licking from selected rocks, an adequate amount to replenish those minerals used, and sufficient for storage in the body against need, should have been obtained. The amounts stored are usually sufficient to service requirements for 6–12 months, but this time span will depend on the current situation of individual animals, for example, pregnant mares will continue to seek calcium and phosphorus which are essential to lactation.

The desert-raised Arabian and the horses of the Steppes living alongside human family groups have their diets supplemented by being fed milk from ewes or camels; dates, both green or ripe, are also included in the Arab diet.

Horses who, when turned out to grass dig soil and begin to eat the dirt, eat their droppings, chew bark, chew fences, are seeking nutrients which they instinctively realise are lacking in their system. If this behaviour is observed, there are several approaches which might be helpful. The first, talking to local farmers who keep stock, who will be able to advise on the supplements they need to feed; second, a soil test may be useful in determining the local mineral profile; and/or third, a test to establish the mineral profile of the individual horse, this can be established by hair analysis.

Does a horse kept naturally need probiotics, indeed, do any of us really need to change a gut flora that has evolved, apparently successfully, over millions of years? One thing is quite certain, most horses are grossly over supplemented.

Many reports indicate that some of the best equine athletes are fed a very simple diet, one consisting of good hay, free range grazing and good quality oats or corn. A recent example confirms this. An endurance horse was continuously unwell for two seasons, despite every additive, balanced feeds and supplementation the animal tied up, was muscle sore, appeared tired, thin, undernourished, had scant, bad-smelling urine and failed every vet check at competition.

It was suggested that the animal be trained from the field, and its diet radically changed, by being simplified. This was done and, in addition to free grazing, carrots and good quality chaff were offered three times a day with an added mineral mix supplement once a week. Rock salt was left at the water trough, a level tablespoon of copper sulphate was added to the field trough if there were any signs of green algae (this worked out at a level tablespoon per month if it was very sunny, less as the ambient temperature got colder). The addition of copper sulphate is an old remedy for keeping field troughs algae free, described in early farming books from the 1800s and before. It allowed the horse access to minute amounts of copper, an element essential for efficient respiratory function.

Within three months the horse was a changed animal. It was bright, alert, well muscled, and as results showed, was competing to a high performance level. In six months the animal was unrecognisable and the rider was being asked where she had found such a marvellous new horse.

After the change in diet, the horse in question covered 725 miles in long-distance competition and was trained 100 miles a week. The animal gained his 1000-mile award, was runner up in three major trophy races and was third in two others. The owner has stated that she was frightened to tell the vets what the animal was being fed as so many of the other horses she was beating were on high-performance rations and she felt it would count against her as a competent keeper if she confessed to such a simple diet.

Nutrition from the ground

All early farming books contained chapters on soil management, for nutrition begins at ground level and every owner should appreciate this. The fact that the grass looks nice and green is no indication of the nutritional value for horses turned out on it. Soil varies from area to area, and depends to a large degree upon the underlying geological strata.

Soil has developed as result of the weathering of ancient rocks and the balance of its contents is secondary to the local rock characteristics; for example, coastal-derived soils, the chalks, contain a high level of calcium collected from the skeletons of ancient marine life.

Another type of valuable precipitate, 30 million years old, is a siliceous mineral compound known as diatomaceous earth (DE); derived from the fossilised pre-historic remains of tiny water algae. Microscopic skeletal remnants of these unicellular plants, called diatoms, appear as a chalk-like deposit in various parts of the world. In Ireland, there is deposit in the Lower Bann Valley, called Bann Clay. Similar characteristics are found in Green Sand, seams of sand-like loam, found in small, localised areas often adjacent to or intermingling with deposits of Fullers Earth.

DE is known to contain 19% calcium, 33% silicon, 5% sodium, 2% iron, as well as many vital trace minerals. There are two sources of DE, that derived from freshwater algae and that from saltwater algae, the latter composed of a highly crystalline form of silica.

It is the sharp, razor-like edges of the silica crystals, that are currently arousing interest as a method of worming. While not yet scientifically proven, the suggestion is the worm larvae in the gut are damaged when they come into contact with the sharp edges of the silica crystals.

One owner, Phil Middleton of Equine America, has recorded worm counts, taken regularly from the faeces samples from a number of his own horses in this country and his partners in the USA over a three-year period. Other than for tape worm, the samples have shown no evidence of worm invasion in the horses fed DE as a supplement.

All soils originally had an individual chemical profile, unfortunately where chemical fertilisation has taken place this has changed most of the original profiles.

Diana Lee has been a researcher and advocate for holistic health solutions for animals and humans since 1984. She has over 200 years of sustainable farming history in her ancestry and considers 'we are now living in a world where soils are depleted by being chemically treated'. The result must be chronic trace mineral deficiencies, and these may well impact health parameters, but unfortunately clinical signs do not usually become apparent until the animal is in an acute deficiency state. There is also an intricate balance between varied elements, high levels of one interfering with absorption of another.

An American publication, *Equine Supplements and Nutraceuticals* (Kellon 1998), provides a comprehensive survey of equine nutritional requirements, discusses plant sources, soil structure, lists the required minerals and vitamins, and describes the effects on the health of the horse in cases of both excess and deficiency. *Nutrient Requirements for Horses* is also a useful source of information but neither publication suggests how to restore denuded soil.

A *Geological Survey of England and Wales* was first published in 1835, and an updated *The Wolfson Geochemical Atlas of England and Wales* based on the work of Professor Webb was published in 1977. The Webb atlas mapped the presence or absence of the chemical elements in each area of England, and also mapped the types of geological substrata. This kind of information gives an idea of the mineral wealth or mineral lack, in all areas, allowing those interested to appreciate the reason for some areas of the country appearing, for example, to be better than others for the growth of young horses, or the reason why hay from a neighbouring county apparently seems to be more nutritious than home-grown hay.

Analysis relating to soil components is carried out by the British Geological Survey Association, Soil Resources, DEFRA and other similar organisations, all of whom will undertake and who publish soil surveys making it possible to detect missing elements. Soil and water analysis are well worth the expenditure. It then only remains to find an expert on soil reconstruction! (See Useful addresses section, page 234.)

It is important to understand soil, because each plant type, even different varieties of grass, vary in their individual requirements in order to complete their lifecycle. Each plant type draws its own, selected minerals from the soil. If the minerals required are not present where the plant is grown, the plant will still grow, but it will be deficient in those minerals it would normally absorb because of their absence from the soil.

One of the most interesting features when regarding nutrition as a whole, is that only *very small* amounts of trace elements and vitamins are needed by the living body, *provided they are obtained from natural sources*. There is no need to debate or even question the fact that the planet on which we live is fully stocked to cater for all our needs. Unfortunately, we have either become too lazy or have forgotten how to seek, grow, prepare and use these natural resources.

Synthetic substitutes, invented by man, have no natural planetary niche and today we face problems which could not have occurred naturally and for which we have no solutions. Chemicals need more chemicals to destroy them; they are not biologically degradable. Such synthetic substances are alien to planetary ecology, there is no mode of recycling as with the natural substances used in the 'pre-pollution' era.

A simple hair analysis (see Table 4.1) will provide a profile of elements present in an individual horse, and it is interesting to note the variations within a group, even though all are receiving the same nutritional base.

Analysis requires a gram of body hair, not taken from the mane or tail, which must be cut with scissors to avoid contamination of oil from clippers. From the sample in Table 4.1, the presence of calcium, magnesium, phosphorus, potassium, sodium, sulphur, iron, manganese, copper, zinc, selenium, arsenic and lead is assayed, the printout showing the levels of each element as low, mean, high or very high.

Nurturing soil

The word *permaculture* is derived from the term 'permanent agriculture' and denotes a self-sustaining agricultural system. The science of agriculture, the means by which essential raw materials for the perpetuation of life in all species are provided, is of paramount importance. To achieve permaculture multi-crop of vegetation is required, which must include annual and perennial plants, mineral-rich, non-compacted soil, water, air and

Table 4.1 An analysis report from a hair sample.

HAIR MINERAL ANALYSIS REPORT

Distributor						Sample No: **H210**		
Farmer:	**Mary. W. Bromiley**							
Sample Ref: **F**					Date:	**23 April 2001**		
Element		Unit	ASSAY	LOW		MEAN	HIGH	VERY HIGH
Calcium	Ca	mg/l	**2363**	0 1000		2000	5000	10000
Magnesium	Mg	mg/l	**1156**	0 250		500	1000	3000
Phosphorus	P	mg/l	**335**	0 100		250	500	1000
Potassium	K	mg/l	**10843**	0 2000		5000	10000	50000
Sodium	Na	mg/l	**2170**	0 1000		3000	7500	25000
Sulphur	S	%	**3.60**	0 1		3	5	10
Iron	Fe	mg/l	**47.80**	0 100		200	500	1000
Manganese	Mn	mg/l	**13.50**	0 5		10	25	50
Copper	Cu	mg/l	**7.30**	0 5		10	20	50
Zinc	Zn	mg/l	**133.00**	0 150		250	500	1000
Selenium	Se	mg/l	**0.43**	0 0.5		0.75	1	5
Arsenic	As	mg/l	**0.17**	0 0.1		1	5	10
Lead	Pb	mg/l	**0.28**	0 1		5	10	50

COMMENTS

Hair Analysis Comments – Sample No: H210
The overall mineral status of this sample follows the pattern set by previous samples in
that a generally high macro-mineral composition is contrasted by a lower range of trace
elements. In this case the potassium: sodium ratio is more appropriate for a healthy
metabolism, although magnesium again dominates the profile. Trace element deficiencies
of iron, zinc and selenium are again suspected, although heavy metal intake is not implicated
in any physiological problems.

animals. The plants, including trees since deciduous trees return nutrients to the soil
each year in the autumn when they drop their leaves, must complement each other's
growth requirements and be appropriate for both the soil and climatic conditions of the
growing area, be it garden or pasture.

The traditional method of retaining healthy soil in the past was through crop rotation, each crop both giving to, as well as taking from the soil bed. Before the intensive,
chemical-based farming of today, animals were turned into fields when the area was
down to grass, or in the case of sheep, planted with turnips; the stock returned nutrients,
via their dung, to the soil while grazing. Mixed, rotted animal manure, spread annually,
topped up requirements.

The texture of the soil is very important. Soils which have become compacted do not
drain and the rootlets of plants may be unable to penetrate the subsoil in order to reach the
deeper, mineral-rich layers. Compaction tends to be the result of heavy farm machinery

and needs to be addressed. The root systems of the plants and earthworms help maintain soil structure naturally but they are unable to cope with compaction. The author
well remembers the day when, following soil analysis after a move, the report stated
'you have sick worms'. The soil had become so compacted over the years that the worms
were confined to the topmost layer; they were small, pale, skinny and useless, neither
breaking down the soil nor available as a nutritious food source for moles, frogs, birds.
The use of a rotary cultivator solved the problem; within a year both worms and soil had
recovered.

It is interesting to note the remarks published in a letter in *Country Life* (03/05/2007)
where the writer describes no-till crop production, a method currently practised by some
farmers in a rocky section of New York State, USA. It involves growing crops without
tillage. The writer states:

> *'as well as eliminating a huge job, turning the soil naturally with horses, this involv-*
> *ing walking 11 miles per acre, the ground improves, with increasing worm pro-*
> *duction and fewer surface stones, as these remain below the surface aiding drainage*
> *instead of being ploughed up annually. Crops thrive on the well-textured soil'.*

There is an interesting picture hung in a museum in Nogales, State of Arizona, USA,
which supports this approach, The picture depicts a native American sitting on his horse
looking down at a settler struggling with a plough. The caption reads 'Why are you turning the ground the wrong way up?' The idea of no till is not new.

Herbs for fodder

Why is it necessary to consider the soil below the grasses eaten by our horse? How does
understanding soil improve our natural horse husbandry? Why should we consider
herbs?

In a natural environment, the horse eats bushes, local plants, most classified as herbs,
rather than grass. The animal is an herbivore not a ruminant. What should we know
about herbs?

Herbs are plants which contain nutrients required by other life forms. Drawing from
and using components present in sunlight, air, water and soil, green plants become the
factories for the production of carbohydrates, fats, proteins, vitamins, and all other
required metabolic compounds necessary for the lives of those that eat the plants.

It is known plants also synthesise non-metabolic compounds; known as secondary
compounds these appear to be of a medicinal nature.

The Romans introduced around 400 species of herb to northern Europe, but the
knowledge of their attributes and properties, both *medicinal* and for the *maintenance* of
general health, stretches back thousands of years.

Many previously unproven attributes of these plants, for example as above, *maintenance* and *medicinal* have now been shown to be correct. To date, around one hundred
thousand different, secondary, plant-manufactured compounds have been identified.

To most of us 'medicine' means the science of healing *after* catastrophe, however, in
the ancient Chinese civilisation, physicians were only paid if their patients stayed
healthy. Surprisingly, the latest edition of Chambers English Dictionary states: 'medicine
is the science or practice of the *prevention* of disease; also of non-surgical methods of
treatment following a diagnosed problem'.

There is evidence of a *Herbal* composed in China around 2700 BC and medical prescriptions were in use and recorded in writing in Egypt around 1800 BC. Even though
minerals are mentioned in these writings, $5/6$ of the recommended ingredients are herbal

in origin. The lore of plant gathering, growing, preserving and the use of roots, followed complex rituals handed down from family member to family member.

This tradition still survives in remote areas and when searching for genuine herbal information, I have often been told that the present 'healer' learnt the secrets from 'pa' who 'had it from his ma' and so on, with five or six past generations often quoted.

Health

Prevention rather than cure is still, as in ancient times, the message of herbalists. The use of herbs is therefore primarily aimed at promoting or maintaining total health.

What do we mean by health? It is a state in which an entire cellular mass, or the mass of cell structures combined to form a recognisable named species, is in a state of harmony, when:

- all the necessary ingredients are present;
- all the storage chambers are filled;
- all the internal organs complement each other's activities;
- all the systems are running smoothly;
- the blood and oxygen are correctly balanced;
- the body mass is fuelled to meet the demands of a workload determined by the level of daily activity;
- the fluid levels and acid–base balance are accurate for the species.

To achieve and maintain this state imposes a need to continually rebuild, replenish and restore. These activities demand the availability of easily assimilated nutrients. Minerals, vitamins and salts from natural sources require the expenditure of less body energy to refine, synthesise and extract than do the man-made chemical substitutes, most of which have unwanted, often detrimental, side effects.

Additives

The horseman of today is bombarded with new products claiming to make the horse 'go faster', 'grow hoof', 'shine coat', 'avoid fatigue' and 'perform better'. There are 'feed mixes', 'feed supplements' and 'feed additives', all of which extol their own particular virtues. After all, the power of advertising is subtle one-upmanship!

Before purchase however, stand back and consider, lest hard earned cash goes in at one end of your horse and comes out at the other. Think logically, how *can* an additive 'reduce oxygen requirements'? It is a scientific impossibility!

Look at the natural requirements of the horse and try to supply these by using nature's ability to manufacture, rather than using man-made chemical replacements. This may require careful soil manipulation. There are natural sources of soil boosting, seaweed being one, but soil correction is the job of an expert and the organic institutions have plenty of advice on offer. Soil cannot be restored instantly. It takes years rather than weeks to recover.

Old (natural) additives

Copper: to ensure adequate copper, important for the development of bones, joints, tendons, ligaments, in areas where copper was known to be deficient, placing a strip of old copper pipe in the water tank was common practice.

Copper sulphate is sometimes used to reduce the formation of green algae in water troughs and acts as a soluble form of copper supplementation. *However*, you must have both a water and soil analysis done to avoid over supplementation.

Root vegetables: the mangold-wurzel (sadly, now rarely grown), turnips, swedes, and carrots, were fed, not as in the case of carrots today as 'treats', but as a valuable, recognised, source of minerals. (All root vegetables store/contain minerals in their root structure rather than in their foliage.)

Turfs: in order to keep the animal healthy, when the horse was an agricultural necessity, it was common practice to cut a sod of turf and place this in the water bucket; water-soluble nutrients are easily absorbed and if not required, easily excreted.

Bran mash: mashes were made by placing an appropriate amount of bran, usually two heaped scoops per horse, into a large container and pouring on sufficient boiling water to thoroughly damp the bran, then the container was put to one side of the tack room stove covered with a cloth and left for several hours.

Mashes were given in place of the evening feed, sometimes after a day of hard work, mostly on Sunday evenings. When the horse was a necessity, a Sunday mash was routine, for other than the Parson's cob, or in an emergency, the trap pony of the local doctor, all horses had a day of rest.

Salt: rock salt sold in large lumps was kept in mangers. If salt was not present in this form, a tablespoon of salt was added when a bran mash was measured out for each individual horse.

Linseed tea: linseed jelly or tea, was made by boiling linseed (the seeds) for at least 6 hours, usually in a double saucepan. When this type of feeding was routine, most tack rooms were warmed by a coke-burning, pot-bellied, stove, ideal for slow cooking.

The jelly was poured off, and an approximate cupful mixed into each mash.

Electrolytes: in some yards when horses returned sweating, the sweat was scraped off into a bucket of luke-warm water, this was then offered to the horse. The stud grooms, whose wisdom was passed down by word of mouth, would never have heard of electrolyte replacement, but that is exactly what they was doing, replacing electrolytes by offering those still present in the sweat in a nice, warm drink. The source of this information (now 92 years old) stated he had never known a horse refuse the drink if offered. (See section on Minerals in Chapter 5, pages 43–45)

Diatomaceous earth: evidence shows that feral animals seek out these sources and lick the area or eat the earth (see www.eqineamerica.co.uk).

Further reading

Davies, B., Eagle, D. & Finney, B. *Soil Management*, 5th edn, Farming Press, Ipswich, 1993

Engel, C. *Wild Health*, Phoenix Orion Books, London, 2002

Holistic Horse, Vols 13–51, 2007, available from *www.holistichorse.com*

Kellon, E.M. *Equine Supplementation and Nutraceuticals*, Breakthrough Publications, New York, 1998

Scamell, J. *Ground Level Nutrition*, available at *jo.scamell@binternet.com*

Stephens, H. *The Book of the Farm*, Vols I & II, 2nd edn, William Blackwood, Edinburgh, 1851

Webb, J.S. (Ed.), *The Wolfson Geochemical Atlas of England and Wales*, Oxford University Press, 1978

5 Feeding

The natural horse eats and drinks head down, it is anatomically designed to do this and when eating in this way the production of saliva is not compromised. Head down, the horse cannot bolt its food and it is forced to chew correctly to assist in the movement of food from the lower area of the mouth, upward, to the entrance of the oesophagus. The head-down position also ensures the food is saturated with saliva during the lengthy process of correct chewing. This is important, for saliva not only makes swallowing easier but it also buffers the gastric acid present in the stomach. If the internal lining of the stomach, the gastric mucosa, is not sufficiently protected from gastric acid, damage can occur, in some cases leading to gastric ulceration. Interestingly gastric ulceration is most common in stabled animals; it is not confined to the racing thoroughbreds as is often commonly supposed, but has been identified in many other disciplines. Research has shown that the amount of saliva produced for each kilogram of concentrate feed is approximately 2.5 times less than an equivalent weight in herbage. The former requires minimal chewing, the latter considerable chewing.

Until relatively recently no yard was without a chaff cutter and all feeds were bulked by the inclusion of *low quality* chaff or chop, the name varying in different parts of the country. This type of *low quality* bulk resulted in correct chewing and increased the volume of ingested matter, allowing the digestive processes to operate normally as they would in the naturally grazing animal, which, reliant on the continual intake of forage to service dietary requirements, eats large quantities of mixed quality herbage.

Ideally, stabled horses should be pastured daily, preferably on an old ley surrounded by natural hedges, forming an environment rich in different plants. Horses have not yet lost their natural ability to choose plants containing the vitamins and minerals which they instinctively appreciate they lack. The ability of the horse to 'doctor' itself is well illustrated by the fact that known 'bleeders' will eat plantains where available, a herb used for haemorrhage control in human herbal remedies. In a free-grazing situation, horses will help themselves, not gorging but nipping a leaf off this, a stem off that – remember minute amounts rebalance systems. They find things in old hedgerows and will often grab at herbage when out hacking. Not bad manners rather 'that is just what I need'.

To appreciate the necessity for a correct balance of components, consider baking a cake; an excess of one ingredient or reduction of another results in failure. The body is no different and problems arise if the addition of additives is not considered in the broadest sense. It is important to know the components of the local soil, to record which 'herbs' (plants) grow at varied times during the seasons, to know what each variety should contain.

Before rushing into designing and planting a herb garden it is sensible to have your soil analysed, then to study the needs of your horse, taking into account workload, season, age and breed. Each of these factors will modify the intake requirement, and as it is exceptionally difficult to achieve the correct balance, it is preferable to allow natural selection by the animal, particularly as most herbs are not 'single suppliers'. For instance

garlic (which can be found growing wild) is a source of antibacterial substances and contains vitamins A, B_1, B_2 and C. The onion is rich in vitamins A, B_1, B_2, C and E. Chives, a
cousin of both garlic and the onion, are easy to grow and a few chopped are not unpalat-
able (see Herbs and their contents, pages 48–68).

To change from a 'prepared' feed, which supposedly contains all the essentials, and to
search for, and feed a balanced diet meeting all requirements using plants obtained from
nature is very time-consuming. Unfortunately, natural supplementation tends to be an
'all or nothing regime'. It cannot be a half-and-half situation, for if you supplement by
allowing your horse to graze and then add artificial supplements 'in case factor X is missing' you are more likely to create problems than to reduce them.

If you buy a new horse try to continue the same feed regime as that of the previous
owner. You may not agree with the previous feeding but find out the routine and change
it slowly.

If you buy a puppy, pedigree, or otherwise, it usually comes with a diet sheet; your
new horse has moved homes, it may be distressed, the food offered is quite different, as
is, in many cases, the water, and it may not eat or drink. Offering food it is used to makes
all the difference.

Nutrition, or the science of feeding

Nutritional experts can only be expected to offer guidelines. It is quite impossible to gen-
eralise a feed programme as each animal, just as each human, has characteristics common to its genetic background.

For the average horse the essential requirements are a balance containing:

- water;
- protein;
- carbohydrate;
- fat;
- minerals;
- vitamins;
- unpolluted air.

Functions of the nutrients

Water

Water is essential for all metabolic processes. Water deficiency is very serious and even
though daily intake will vary, a horse needs access to fresh water at all times. When away
from home, for example at a competition, it is advisable to take home water for the
horse to drink.

Water is lost:

- during the excretion of urine;
- in the faeces;
- when sweating;
- via respiratory evaporation during expiration.

The amount of dry matter fed will also influence the daily water requirements. If your
horse has to be stabled it should be noted that metal, self-filling drinking bowls can, in
frosty conditions become very cold. It seems ridiculous that horses can become dehy-

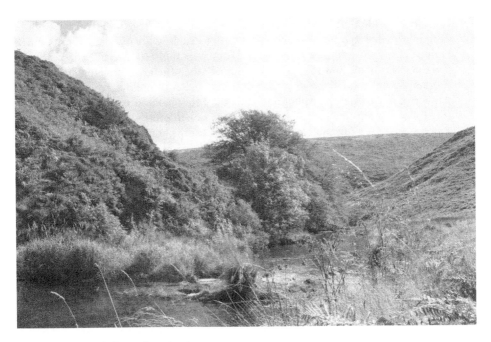

Fig. 5.1 A stream is the preferred water source.

drated in cold weather but they do, as they are unable to tolerate icy water. It is well worth offering water to the horse stabled or otherwise, with the chill taken off by the addition of hot water in cold conditions.

Horses often enjoy drinking from streams (see Fig. 5.1) and ponds rather than from a bucket put into the field. This should not be discouraged as most streams carry dissolved minerals, and some horses dislike the 'man-made additives/pollutants' included in tap water. Of these, nitrates and fluoride are the least tolerated, both are under scrutiny from EU regulations involving water quality.

An article published in the *Journal for International Research*, (2006), reported signs of fluoride poisoning in a group of Quarter horses. While cattle and sheep are known to be affected by fluoride, very little research has been undertaken to date in horses.

Nitrate can be converted in the caecum of the horse to nitrite. Nitrite unfortunately interferes with the transport of oxygen by displacing oxygen on the haemoglobin molecule forming methaemoglobin, which in turn reduces oxygen transport to the tissues.

Protein

Amino acids, some of which are synthesised by the body, with others obtained from external sources, constitute the fundamental structure of all proteins. Proteins form the structural material of the tissues, the muscles and the body organs, and they are important regulators of function, in common with enzymes and hormones.

Excess protein, i.e. in amounts in excess of that required by the animal, can be converted into glucose to be stored and used as energy. However, excessive protein intake is *not* beneficial.

As exercise demands increase, leading to the need for tissue repair and remodelling, adjustment of protein intake will be necessary, but the exact amount will require consideration. You may choose to address the increased need by introducing hay containing a higher protein level or by increasing the levels in hard feed. In all cases, any increase should be gradual. It is worth remembering that any change of hay, haylage or similar bulking foods require careful consideration as each will vary widely in its nutritional value. These variations depend on the source of the feed, the time of year when the product was made and the moisture content when the grasses were cut. Far too many horses 'tie up' following the arrival of a new batch of bulking feed. In the days when sufficient hay to last the winter and enough of that batch was still in the barn to be fed the following autumn, a base of similar nutritional levels was maintained, the hay was never 'too rich'. Constant changes are difficult for the horse to adapt to and create digestive problems, which lead in turn to loss of condition and reduced performance levels.

While considering protein intake it follows that if exercise demands decrease, so protein levels should be reduced. Overfeeding, using high quality feeds, is often more disastrous than giving slightly less. The most important factor for the horse is always to have adequate, good quality feed, which is free of both dust and moulds. These are not confined to hay alone, oats get musty in damp conditions, as do all bagged balanced ration feeds, even carrots.

Carbohydrate

Energy sources required for muscle activity are drawn from the conversion of the carbohydrate chain of sugars present in the fibre of the horse's food. In the natural horse, the primary source of energy in equine diet is culled from the carbohydrate intake. This energy is absorbed from the intestine as glucose, and any excess not immediately required is stored as glycogen both in muscle and in the liver. The muscle store is ready for immediate use on demand, the glycogen stored in the liver is available as a 'back up', released into the blood stream when required, to be rapidly transported to areas of need.

Bulky feeding, natural or otherwise, is important due to the design of the equine digestive system and the in-built requirement of the horse to chew. Well-bulked food, if grazing is supplemented, with the concentrates mixed with chop (chaff), will encourage the horse to chew slowly, grinding the food matter and ensuring an efficient start to the general digestive process and subsequent metabolic absorption. It has been calculated that a kilo of bulked food will require the horse to chew approximately 5,300 times, whereas a kilo of concentrates will only be chewed around 1,000 times, the latter creating a bolus or block of food, which passes rapidly first into the stomach and then into the intestines rather than achieving the required continual, steady, delivery flow, achieved by the slow passage of bulked food as in the grazing/browsing animal.

Fats and/or oils

Some confusion exists regarding terminology: fats and oils are both lipids, the main difference being their state. The term fat refers to a compound which is solid at room temperature, while oils are liquid. There is a body requirement for lipids in feeds, particularly as the body is unable to synthesise certain types of fatty acids.

While the requirement for a supply of lipids is not entirely energy based, horses can use fats as an energy source during prolonged aerobic muscle work. Appropriate fats also provide a highly concentrated source of energy able to supply twice the number of calories, weight for weight, when compared with carbohydrates. The exercise demands of the horse must be assessed prior to increasing the fat ration as fats are *not* a substitute for carbohydrate. The feeding levels of acceptable fats as a source of increased dietary energy needs expert advice. Horses in a natural state, where the compounds are obtained from vegetation seem to require around 3% lipids in the diet. In man-offered rations, corn and sunflower oils are two sources of acceptable fat and, being plant derived, are easily utilised by the horse; fish oil has a different molecular structure and while the horse is able to digest plant-derived lipids easily, fish oil seems of doubtful use. Horses do not try to catch fish as a source of nutrition, bears do!

Minerals

Minerals are inorganic elements, processed mainly via plants, which when ingested deliver the minerals they carry to their host. Minerals are essential ingredients for health, those assisting in the regulation/maintenance of body fluids are termed *electrolytes*. Calcium, phosphorus, potassium, sodium, chloride, magnesium and sulphur are all required in reasonable amounts. Iron, copper, cobalt, iodine, manganese and zinc are needed in lesser amounts, with only minute amounts of selenium required.

Minerals are involved in:

- energy transfer;
- fluid balance;
- maintenance of osmotic pressure;
- activity within both the nervous and muscular systems;
- they also assist in forming many of the body structures.

Mineral loss

The horse does not manufacture minerals, they must be obtained through feed. Electrolytes deserve explanation. An electrolyte is a pure mineral element capable of carrying an electrical charge which may be positive or negative. When dissolved, the resultant solution created will conduct electrical signals, thus assisting in internal communication.

While a wide range of minerals required to sustain life is involved in a variety of functions, some are of particular importance in maintaining the correct fluid balance within the body. Unfortunately, when considering the regulation of body fluids, over supplementation does not help, as the body is unable to store the appropriate electrolytes against need. This is due to the fact that the body must retain an electrolytic balance appropriate to maintain a normal fluid balance.

Indiscriminate loading also has a tendency to interfere with normal absorption, thus some minerals, even though present can become 'locked up' and are therefore unavailable to the horse.

Horses lose minerals/electrolytes in significant amounts in their sweat. If there has been a significant loss of some minerals, for example potassium and sodium chloride and they are not available in feed, these will need to be replaced, either by an electrolyte supplement, preferably administered in water if the horse will drink, by drenching if it will not drink, or as a powder. Unfortunately, electrolytes need to be suspended in fluid before they can pass from the intestines into the body mass, so when administered in liquid form they are rapidly absorbed, in a powder form the digestive system must make fluid available for suspension, often, if the horse is dehydrated, at some cost.

In cases of extreme exhaustion replacement necessitates veterinary intervention, replacement effected through a saline drip.

Minerals and their uses

Calcium

- Required for the development of bones and teeth.
- Required for muscle contraction.
- Required for the transmission of nerve impulses (messages).
- Involved in the maintenance of the rhythm of the heart.
- Involved in cell membrane permeability.

Chlorine

- Involved in the digestive process in the stomach.
- Assists in the acid–base balance.
- Is the main anion in extracellular fluid.
- Assists in the preparation of chemical energy.
- Assists in protein synthesis.

Copper

- Involved in the synthesis and absorption of iron to perfect haemoglobin.
- Involved in electron transport.
- Involved in the construction of nerve insulation (sheath).

Fluorine

- Required to prevent decay in bones and teeth.

Iron

- Required for the formation of haemoglobin and myoglobin.
- A constituent of oxidative enzymes.

Magnesium

- Required for muscle and nerve response (irritability).
- Required for carbohydrate metabolism.
- A constituent of teeth and bone.

Manganese

- Involved in the formation of bone.
- Required for bone and tooth formation.
- Required for cell permeability.
- Involved in activating the enzyme activity for many processes.

Phosphorus

- Required for the metabolism of carbohydrates and fats.
- Involved in the storage and release of ATP (adenosine triphosphate).

Potassium

- Required for response of nerve and muscle to commands.
- Is the principal cation of the intracellular fluid.
- Involved in both water and acid–base balance.
- Involved in maintenance of heart rhythm.
- Involved in protein synthesis.

Selenium

- An antioxidant.
- Excess is toxic.

Sodium

- Involved in the regulation of nerve irritability.
- Involved in the regulation of muscle contraction.
- Involved in both water and the acid–base balance.
- The principal cation in extracellular fluid.

Sulphur

- A vital constituent of proteins, especially important in cartilage.
- Involved in detoxification.
- A necessary constituent for many complex interactions.

Zinc

- A vital constituent of enzymes.
- Necessary for the completion of many complex body interactions.

Vitamins

Vitamins are complex organic compounds, micronutrients which are essential for health. Some are manufactured by the body, but once again plants supply the majority of the body's needs. Plant tissue manufactures vitamins during its growing cycle, and different plants or 'herbage' supply variable quantities and categories of vitamins.

Lack of vitamins or an incorrect balance gives rise to conditions classed as deficiency diseases. Beriberi (caused by vitamin B deficiency) was described as early as 2600 BC in China. No 'cure' was found, or none was recorded, until 1880 – nearly 5000 years later. A reduction in the incidence of the disease was noticed when in the late eighteen hundreds brown rice replaced highly milled (polished) rice on board Japanese naval ships. The fact that polishing the rice removed the outer thiamine-rich (vitamin B) covering or 'coat' of the grains was recorded by Jansen & Donath in 1926 (Mervyn 1984).

Preference for natural sources is obvious – the body has developed and evolved within its environment and all elements within its structure are naturally adapted to assimilate plant-produced nutrients. Body components do not easily recognise synthetic products and are often unable to use or ingest them, with many merely excreted, having been classified as 'incompatible'.

As stated earlier, natural herbage and grains contain the most vitamins, but the herbage must be of good quality. Bleached hay, hay with serious leaf loss, poor quality, stale or mouldy food will all have had their original vitamin content depleted. Horses fed poor quality forage and those which do not have access to pasture and sunlight will require vitamin supplementation, not only in their food, but also by the use of ultraviolet light in a solarium to enable the horse to synthesise vitamin D.

Vitamin D is involved in the metabolism of calcium which is essential not only for bone structure but also for efficient muscle activity. A lack of natural sunlight is serious and horses who suffer this will not be as healthy as those exposed to natural sunlight. In these instances a solarium will go some way to improving health.

Vitamins are sub-divided into two groups: those classified as *water soluble* and those classified as *fat soluble*. For successful reactivity, many vitamins need to interact with one or more minerals. Vitamins were first recognised in 1911, and by 1977 fifteen had been 'discovered'. *The Dictionary of Vitamins* (Mervyn 1984) lists 23 and there are undoubtedly many more as yet unidentified but certainly present, probably both organically and within the body components. As described in the herb vitamin section, vitamins are involved in:

- nerve conductivity;
- all metabolic processes;
- tissue building;
- body defence;
- digestion;
- food assimilation;
- all manufacturing processes.

Each animal should be considered individually and a ration both balanced and appropriate to its needs formulated.

Vitamins and their uses

The following list is of major vitamins, all have known specific functions.

Vitamin A

- Required for absorption.
- Stored in the liver.
- Required for enhancing vision in dim light.
- Maintains the health of certain cells, in particular those lining the airways (the mucosal epithelium).
- Excess is toxic.

Vitamin B_1

- Involved in carbohydrate metabolism.

Vitamin B_2

- Involved in energy metabolism.

Vitamin B_6

- Involved in protein metabolism.

Vitamin B_{12}

- Involved in the formation of red blood cells.
- Involved in energy production, particularly the synthesis of DNA and RNA.

Vitamin C

- Involved in the absorption of iron.

Vitamin D

- Regulates calcium and phosphate metabolism.
- Assists in the mineralisation of bone.

Vitamin E

- Reacts with selenium.
- Regulates calcium and phosphorus absorption.

Vitamin K

- Assists in the formation of essential blood clotting agents.
- Large amounts are toxic.

Sunlight

Before considering the herbal sources of the nutrients required, it is essential to consider in more depth a freely available essential health constituent which has already been mentioned in passing – *sunlight*. As with many notable scientific discoveries the power and necessity of sunlight for health was an accidental discovery. Dr John Ott was a photographer, his specialty being time-lapse photography. After many years of experimenting he realised that some light rays essential for the full growth and fertility of the plants he was photographing were being filtered out by the glass that protected the plants, so he turned to assessing the effects on laboratory animals of lack of light, and exposure to varying light wave lengths. He came to realise that the full spectrum of daylight was essential for harmonious living.

Much has been written about the nutritional requirements of animals and humans. The complex role played by natural minerals and vitamins is continually being unravelled, but the need for one vital commodity is rarely, if ever, mentioned – that commodity is *sunlight*. All energy is derived in some manner from the sun. Consider plants which *photosynthesise* or absorb sunlight to create the energy they require to live, grow and reproduce. The green colour of plants arises from chlorophyll. Molecules of chlorophyll are able to absorb sunlight and in a complex chain reaction, combine with water and carbon dioxide to create carbohydrates – the 'food' from which the plant derives the energy for its complex life pattern. During the conversion of absorbed sunlight into carbohydrate, oxygen is created and released to the atmosphere. The animal kingdom consumes varied species of plant, their seeds or fruit, selecting, by intuition, those required. This a natural method of nutritional uptake.

The consumer's body then extracts the nutrients it requires and slowly, a complex cycle (Kreb's cycle) breaks down the carbohydrate content, extracting energy and using that energy as and where it is needed and/or required, from each step of Kreb's cycle. The process eventually reforms the original water and carbon dioxide, both of which are excreted in re-usable forms thereby completing the 'natural cycle'.

Plants and animals have co-existed since animal life initially evolved. The sun was here first, then plants developed, followed by the animal kingdom. Today, in the twenty-first century, our lives are very different from those of our ancestors, who lived a more 'natural' existence: we shut ourselves from the sun and have even become fearful of its effect upon us. However, it is the way we use the sun rather than the sun itself that does the harm. Gentle exposure encourages the production of the chemical melanin; melanin darkens the skin and ensures protection from the damaging rays. The world's human population adapted to climatic conditions, with dark-skinned people near the equator and light-skinned people away from the equator. Dark skins filter out damaging rays and light skins allow absorption in areas where the sunlight is less caustic.

There are shade-loving plants, plants which prefer light from the north and full sun lovers; site a plant in a situation for which it is not suited and it is unlikely to thrive; over-exposure is as harmful as underexposure.

In today's world many domestic animals spend more and more time indoors screened from sunlight. Boxes may be in a barn, shaded by an overhang, grills on doors prevent the animal from putting its head outside its box and many horses spend as much as 23 hours out of every 24 in their boxes. Even those turned out wear screening New Zealand rugs. They are being starved of an ingredient vital for the metabolic activities of calcium and phosphorus – the correct absorption in the intestine, retention and mobilisation. It makes little difference if a formulated diet contains calcium and phosphorus in the assumed correct ratio, unless the 'sunshine vitamin' (vitamin D) is present problems are inevitable.

How does an animal get vitamin D? Unfortunately, the distribution of vitamin D in herbage is poor. Some is formed when certain pasture species begin to fade, provided they are exposed to sunlight at the time. The ideal time for that exposure is the two hours either side of midday – early morning sun or late afternoon sun will have less effect. Lack of natural vitamin D presupposes that sunlight is never in short supply, for the body manufactures vitamin D in response to exposure to sunlight.

Life requires many things to sustain it. Through the millennia different species have adapted to their native environmental conditions. They may be smaller in size if they have less sun but nevertheless they have adapted. Problems begin when species are moved to different environmental conditions, particularly if these movements occur at critical developmental stages in the animal's life. Air travel has made the transportation of the horse a commonplace event. For example, an animal roams the pastures in New Zealand at a formative phase of its development. It is making use of a wide range of mineral- and vitamin-rich herbage and natural water in its development and it has hours of sunlight filtering through an atmosphere free from the levels of pollution seen in the UK. The animal is suddenly transported, over a 36-hour period, to the UK. It is probably stabled on arrival and is therefore *cut off from sunlight*. The feed and water bear no resemblance to those to which its body's metabolic processes are accustomed. If it is an in-foal mare, how can the growing fetus be unaffected by such a catastrophic change?

Abrams in 1978 pointed out that many horses are exercised in the early morning before being housed for the rest of the day, and thus must be lacking essential sunlight.

A problem with any deficiency is that it is rarely immediately apparent. Lack of nutrients in one generation will be rectified by the extraction of the necessary nutrients from the body's stores. Breed from that animal and the next generation will be a shade less robust. The spiral will continue downward until problems such as porous bones, spontaneous fractures, or reduced muscle activity become agonisingly apparent.

If possible, include natural sunlight in your horse's diet – after all, it is a free additive! If a solarium is to be substituted as the source of light, check the bulbs – they must emit full spectrum light to be of value.

For the reader who is thinking 'sun exposure equals skin cancer', *please* substitute '*sunburn* or *skin fry* equals damage'. Traumatise skin and it will react unfavourably. It also follows that an excess of anything, no matter in what context, is bad for any living species. The human race tends to overindulge; animals and plants take what they need. Animals will move out of excess sunlight into shade if it is available and plants are able to operate shut-down mechanisms to protect themselves. Solarium manufacturers should indicate minimum and maximum graded time exposures. *Do not* be tempted to overexpose on the principle that if five minutes is good ten minutes will be better. If your horse is not used to exposure it will take time to adapt.

Herbs for health

Unfortunately, the many changes in the agricultural policies of recent decades have led to the destruction of 'natural' meadows where a variety of different species supported each other. The indiscriminate use of nitrogen has caused massive changes in soil composition and many areas have become practically sterile as intensive cropping has robbed the soil of all components. However, it is perfectly possible to sow and grow many of the common herbs, making certain that the soil is in good heart before planting or sowing. Seaweed is an excellent compound for putting life back into the soil in denuded areas.

It is possible to purchase dried herbs and herb mixes. The bulk amount required will vary, because there is some loss of content when herbs are provided, chopped and dried, rather than being offered fresh. If you 'gather' allow for a loss of 30% of potency. This loss occurs within 24 to 36 hours of gathering. Herbs must be dried correctly and always stored in a cool dry area.

Taste can be an indicator of use. Pleasant tasting herbs are tonic herbs and help maintain health; medical herbs tend to be bitter – not all are edible, some are poisonous, or if their leaves are safe then their roots may not be. Herbalism is a science – to become proficient requires in-depth study.

'There are no known side effects from herbs used knowledgeably and wisely. *Knowledge* and *wisdom* are the key words. Herbs cannot be used indiscriminately without knowledge, no more than can food. We must use common sense, fortified with a basic knowledge of the properties of herbs and an appreciation of body requirements in order to use them effectively.'

Stan Malstrom, *Own Your Own Body* (1988)

The first part of this section has mentioned the bare nutritional requirements of a horse and touches on a very few of the complex interactions and processes involved in the functions of living. This section endeavours to expand the theme by linking vitamins and mineral necessities to herb sources, in rather more depth. The herbs discussed are commonly found growing in the countryside, at the appropriate time of year. Names may vary in countries other than the UK but a botany text should provide adequate cross reference.

Vitamins and minerals are described, their role in body metabolism is suggested, herb sources are recorded and possible deficiency characteristics suggested.

It must be realised that deficiency conditions result from multiple influences, rather than from a single factor.

The term *metabolism* refers to the highly complex and complicated changes the body cells, in their various 'factory systems', achieve using the ingredients delivered to the digestive system in the shape of ingested food. Some of the changes occur as a result of activity by resident intestinal microbial elements, some occur through enzyme activity, some through interaction with cell secretions, some by coupling with minerals, and some by complex chemical reactions.

You will notice that no values are given in following sections of the text headed 'Equine Requirements'. This is because exact values have *not* been established, however it is appreciated that horses do need all the vitamins and minerals listed.

It is obvious from the herb sources mentioned that the natural living, free ranging animal, would have been able to select herbage containing the mineral/vitamin components necessary to sustain life.

Historical uses for herbs

Herbs have been used for many different reasons throughout history, but primarily to maintain health. They have also been used for healing. Herbal lore was passed from healer to acolyte by word of mouth. Before writing was invented no form of early records existed, neither are there reports recording success or failure from those earlier times, unlike the medical statistics of today.

Listed below are some of the purposes for which herbs were/are utilised.

Alternative: Herbs used to change existing nutritious and elimination processes to regulate body functions.
Analgesic: Herbs used to ease pain when taken internally.
Anodyne: Herbs used to ease pain when used externally.
Antibiotic: Herbs used to terminate growth of harmful micro-organisms.
Antihydropic: Herbs used to eliminate excess body fluid.
Anti-inflammatory: Herbs used to reduce inflammation.
Antipyretic: Herbs used to relieve fevers.
Antiseptic: Herbs used to stop, fight and counteract toxic bacteria.
Antispasmodic: Herbs used to sooth contractions or coughing.
Antisyphilitic: Herbs used to relieve venereal diseases.
Aphrodisiac: Herbs used to cure problems of impotency and restore sexual power.
Aromatic: Herbs that have an aromatic taste and stimulate the mucous membrane in the intestines.

Astringent: Herbs used to condense tissues and stop discharges.
Calmative: Herbs used to calm the nervous system.
Cardiac: Herbs used to make the heart stronger.
Carminative: Herbs used to eliminate gas from the digestive system.
Cathartic: Herbs used to encourage purging from the bowel.
Cell proliferant: Herbs used to heal and stimulate new cell growth.
Cholagogue: Herbs to increase flow of bile into the duodenum.
Demulcent: Herbs used to soothe and protect areas which are painful or inflamed
    internally.
Depurant: Herbs used to purify the blood, stimulating the elimination procedures.
Diaphoretic: Herbs used to encourage perspiration.
Digestant: Herbs containing enzymes, amino acids, etc., to help in the digestion of food.
Diuretic: Herb used to increase urine flow.
Emmenagogue: Herbs used to stimulate suppressed menstrual flow.
Emollient: Herbs used to soften and protect the skin.
Expectorant: Herbs used to eliminate toxic mucus from the respiratory system.
Febrifuge: Herbs used to reduce fevers.
Haemostatic: Herbs used to stop bleeding.
Hepatic: Herbs used to strengthen the liver and increase the flow of bile.
Hormonal: Herbs containing hormonal properties.
Laxative: Herbs used as a mild laxative, stimulating bile and secretions rather than irrit-
    ating the bowel.
Mucilaginous: Herbs with an adhering, expanding property, with soothing qualities for
    healing.
Nervine: Herbs used to calm the nerves.
Nutritive: Herbs that are nutritious and encourage growth.
Purgative: Herbs used to cause purging from the bowels, used generally in a combina-
    tion with other herbs to control action.
Relaxant or *Sedative*: Herbs used for their calming properties.
Stimulant: Herbs used to increase the energy levels of the body, or its parts or organs.
Stomachic: Herbs used to strengthen the stomach and encourage the appetite.
Sudorific: Herbs that encourage perspiration.
Tonic: Herbs that stimulate and give the body energy.
Vermicide: Herbs used to kill parasites.
Vermifuge: Herbs used to expel worms.
Vulnerary: Herbs that encourage the healing of wounds.

Vitamins and their herb sources

All books on equine nutrition list vitamins as an essential requirement. Most include at
least short sections on vitamins A, the B family, C, D and E. However, we are still a long
way from a full list and exact requirement values are mostly unknown. You will find
information below on vitamins H, K, P and U, together with PABA. These have been
included not because they appear in equine nutritional literature, but because they are
present in the natural herbage that grows where wild horses lived and therefore must
have formed part of their diet.

References to herb sources pinpoint alfalfa as the most common denominator, with
dandelion not far behind. 'Alfalfa hay', I can hear the cry, 'but remember it will have had
its vitamin content considerably reduced by drying, crushing and through in-leaf loss.
Alfalfa can be grown and fed fresh, and if fertilised with a seaweed preparation, it should

contain all its vitamins and minerals (see section below on Minerals and their herb sources, pages 57–64).

This text should not be taken as dictating proven and definite values. For those interested in formulating diets, the identified mineral and vitamin requirements for the horse can be found by reference to *Equine Supplements and Nutraceuticals* (Kellon 1998).

N.B.: It must be noted that no exact requirement values can be identified in the absence of an analysis of the current feed being used, analysis should always include hard feed, hay, grazing and water. If an animal is allowed free range, free selection and the appropriate herbage is present with the essential nutrients in the soil, the animal will balance its own required intake.

The role each compound plays, the effects associated with deficiency and plant sources are briefly described below.

Commonly found herbs which can be gathered easily, are highlighted in bold type. Their appearance will be seasonal but remember the horse is designed to live in this manner.

Vitamin A (Retinol)

- Fat soluble. Essential for the body to manufacture visual purple (rhodopsin), which is necessary for night vision.
- Vitamin A requires fats as well as minerals to be assimilated. It is an antioxidant. Antioxidants protect other substances from uncontrolled oxidations which damage cells. They help keep pollutants in check. (Antioxidants are vitamins A, C, E and selenium.)
- Associated with:
  - vision;
  - maintenance of normal epithelium (the epithelium lines and protects many body organs including the respiratory and digestive tracts);
  - healthy skin;
  - reproduction;
  - bone development;
  - cartilage integrity;
  - immune responses to disease including respiratory disease.
- Main signs of deficiency:
  - eye disorders;
  - dry, brittle coat;
  - susceptibility to infection;
  - frequent respiratory infections;
  - defective bone modelling.
- Herb sources:
  Alfalfa, Camomile, Comfrey, Dandelion, Fennel, Ginger, Kelp, **Peppermint, Red clover, Rose hips.**

Vitamin B₁ (Thiamine)

- Water soluble. Also called morale or pep vitamins. All B vitamins should be taken as a B complex, i.e. one B alone is useless.
- Associated with:
  - protein and carbohydrate metabolism (Krebs' cycle);
  - digestion;
  - maintenance of normal red blood cell count;
  - muscle tone of heart, intestines and stomach.
- Main signs of deficiency:
  - loss of mental alertness;
  - loss of appetite;
  - respiratory problems;

- heart irregularities;
- fatigue.
- Herb sources:
Alfalfa, Dandelion, Garlic, Hops, Hawthorn, Kelp, **Red clover.**

Vitamin B_2 (Riboflavin)

- Water soluble. Vitamin B_2 is not destroyed by heat, oxidation or acid. There is increased need during stress.
- Associated with:
  - healthy skin, coat, hooves;
  - absorption of iron;
  - utilisation of carbohydrates, fat, protein.
- Main signs of deficiency:
  - digestive disturbances;
  - anaemia;
  - fatigue;
  - poor growth;
  - severe weight loss.
- Herb sources:
Alfalfa, Chickweed, Dandelion, Hops, Hawthorn, Red clover.

Vitamin B_3 (Niacin or Nicotinic Acid, Nicotinamide)

- Water soluble. The body can manufacture its own niacin.
- Associated with:
  - nervous system function;
  - circulation of blood;
  - metabolism of proteins, carbohydrates, fats;
  - cell respiration.
- Main signs of deficiency can include:
  - severe digestive problems.
- Herb sources:
Alfalfa, Dandelion, Hawthorn, Hops, Kelp, **Red clover, Rose hips.**

Vitamin B_5 (Pantothenic Acid)

- Water soluble. It is found in all living cells. It is known as the anti-stress vitamin, and can be produced by naturally occurring bacteria in the intestines.
- Associated with:
  - drug detoxification;
  - chemical transmitted at the synapse of nerve.
- Main signs of deficiency:
  - unknown.
- Herb sources:
Alfalfa, Dandelion, Chickweed, Ginger, Hawthorn, Hops, Red clover.

Vitamin B_6 (Pyridoxamine)

- Immune system building antibodies.
- The metabolism of protein, carbohydrate, fats.
- Wound healing.
- Avoidance of fatigue.
- Water soluble, it is excreted within eight hours of ingestion. Higher amounts are needed during pregnancy and lactation, and with high protein diets.

- Associated with:
  - production of antibodies;
  - DNA and RNA synthesis;
  - haemoglobin synthesis;
  - magnesium assimilation;
  - helps to metabolise fats, carbohydrates and protein;
  - aids in absorption of B_{12};
  - body fluid balance by regulating potassium and sodium levels in the body.
- Main signs of deficiency:
  - impaired ability to utilise glycogen (main muscle fuel);
  - impaired ability to use protein;
  - behaviour changes in mares when in season.
- Natural sources:
  Carrots, molasses, wheat bran
- Herb sources:
  Alfalfa, Dandelion, Ginger, Hops, **Kelp, Red clover.**

Vitamin B_9 (Folicin or Folic Acid)

- Water soluble. Folic acid was named because it is present in the 'foliage' of certain plants.
- Also considered to be the 'other anti-anaemia vitamin'.
- Associated with:
  - synthesis of DNA and RNA;
  - transmission of genetic code;
  - associates with B_{12} to prevent anaemia;
  - disease resistance.
- Main signs of deficiency:
  - poor performance;
  - anaemia.
- Natural sources:
  Root vegetables, carrots, swedes, mangolds, turnips.
- Herb sources:
  Alfalfa, Dandelion, Ginger, **Hawthorn, Hops, Red clover,** Kelp.

Vitamin B_{12} (Cobalamin)

- Water soluble. It is called the red vitamin. Unlike most water-soluble vitamins it can be stored by the body.
- Vitamin B_{12} deficiency is considered to be secondary to a deficiency of cobalt.
- Associations:
  - essential for all basic metabolic processes;
  - excess of dietary protein increases the need for B_{12};
  - increased performance levels increase the need for B_{12}.
- Main signs of deficiency:
  - anaemia;
  - lack of metabolic activity.

N.B.: The identification, B_{12}, is considered by experts in nutrition to represent not one, but rather a complex group of compounds. These compounds are involved in nearly every cell activity and metabolic process.

If B_{12} is lacking, supplementation may need to be by injection. The body may be unable to absorb B_{12} in cases of deficiency and there are no known vegetation sources.

- Natural sources; herb sources:
  - none. Considered to be manufactured in the intestinal tract by micro-organisms.

Vitamin C (Ascorbic Acid)

- Water soluble. The first vitamin discovered by man. It is a cure for scurvy. It needs to be replaced daily; most animals manufacture their own vitamin C. It is an antioxidant and a universal antitoxin, which means it helps protect against harmful oxidation which damages cells, and protects against poisonous and harmful substances of all kinds. It has a primary role in the formation of collagen and helps the body's absorption of iron.
- Considered to be manufactured by animals to service requirements.
- Associated with:
  - collagen synthesis in all tissues;
  - interlinks with B_{12};
  - defence against the invasion of the body by bacterial and viral incidents;
  - improved wound healing;
  - iron metabolism.
- Main signs of deficiency:
  - disturbed collagen metabolism in young animals;
  - poor performance particularly following bacterial or viral invasion;
  - bleeding in lungs at exercise;
  - allergies.
- Natural sources:
  Apples, blackberries.
- Herb sources:
  Alfalfa, Dandelion, Comfrey, Red clover.

B complex Choline

- Choline is considered an essential nutrient for all species, but little else is known about it.
- Manufactured by the animal, probably synthesised in the liver.
- Assists in:
  - the regulation of metabolic process;
  - growth factors;
  - formation of acetylcholine associated with the transmission of nerve impulses;
  - fat metabolism aiding energy production.
- Main signs of deficiency:
  - poor growth;
  - haemorrhage in kidneys;
  - inability to synthesise fat.
- Natural sources:
  Sugar beet, whole oats, wheat bran, soybean (now GM take care).
- Herb sources:
  Alfalfa.

Vitamin D: D_3 (Cholecalciferol) animal; D_2 (Ergocalciferol) plant

- The 'sunshine' vitamin, so called because it can only be manufactured if the body is exposed to sufficient sunlight, the ultraviolet end of the spectrum being the most important. *Unfortunately, many animals are denied sunlight because of modern*

husbandry techniques. Vitamin D has been shown to function as a hormone rather than as a pure vitamin.
- It has been demonstrated that 11 to 45 minutes of daily sunshine prevent vitamin D deficiency manifesting in growing chicks.
- Assists in:
  - mineralisation of bone by acting with calcium and phosphorus;
  - essential for all functions associated with calcium and phosphorus (e.g. muscle activity);
  - concerned with the immune activity of cells;
  - concerned with the recycling of calcium via the kidney.

N.B.: The ratio of calcium to phosphorus is crucial when determining vitamin D requirements. A ratio of 1.2 calcium to 1.0 phosphorus seems to be the requirement of adult stock. If this ratio of 1.2:1.0 changes, becoming narrower or wider, the requirement for vitamin D increases.

- Main signs of deficiency:
  - weak porous bones;
  - enlargement (in young animals) of knee and hock joints;
  - abnormal hyaline cartilage;
  - spontaneous fractures;
  - delayed epiphyseal closure (epiphysitis).
- Sources:
  - sunlight;
  - plants only contain very small amounts of vitamin D and the body has ineffective methods of absorbing the vitamin from plants, presumably because sufficient is produced within the body by exposure to sunlight.

Vitamin E (Tocopherol)

- Fat soluble. Unlike other fat-soluble vitamins it is stored for a short period of time in the body and then any extra is eliminated in the faeces.
- *Tocopherol* is Greek for 'ability to bear young'. Vitamin E's reputation for helping fertility is well known. Selenium associates with vitamin E and increases its power.
- Manganese needs to be present in the body for vitamin E to be effective.
- The oxidation of body cells is the partial cause of ageing. Vitamin E has been used to retard ageing. (Synthetic E will not prevent the oxidation of vitamin A.)
- Blood flow is improved by vitamin E and it causes blood vessels to dilate or expand.
- It is an inhibitor of improper blood coagulation, thus it helps prevent blood clots. It has been called nature's blood thinner. However, unlike chemical blood thinners it does not cause haemorrhage.
- Associated with:
  - antioxidant;
  - cell respiration;
  - inhibits platelet clumping;
  - may work with B_{12};
  - assists in reactions of creatine phosphate and adenosine triphosphate.
- Main signs of deficiency:
  - muscle degeneration;
  - possibly linked to 'tying up' syndrome.
- Herb sources:
  Alfalfa, Comfrey, Dandelion, Linseed, Rose hip, Sunflower.

Vitamin H (Biotin, Coenzyme R)

- Water soluble; member of the B complex family. It is found in small amounts in all living tissue. It can be synthesised by the intestinal bacteria. It is essential to the metabolism of carbohydrates, proteins, fat and unsaturated fatty acids.
- Assists in:
  - metabolism of carbohydrates, protein, fats, especially unsaturated fatty acids;
  - normal growth;
  - maintains healthy skin, sebaceous glands, nerves, and bone marrow;
  - hoof growth.
- Main signs of deficiency:
  - poor hoof growth;
  - fatigue;
  - poor appetite.
- Natural sources:
  Wheat bran, rolled oats.
- Herb sources:
  Alfalfa, Dandelion, Hawthorn, Hops, Kelp, Red clover.

Vitamin K (Phytomenadione)

- Vitamin K is named after the Danish word for blood clotting, *coagulation*.
- It is important in the production of the clotting agent prothrombin and in the conversion of glucose to glycogen (the form of sugar stored in the body for use as fuel).
- Vitamin K is produced in the intestines.
- Assists in:
  - promotes proper blood clotting;
  - reduces haemorrhage.
- Natural sources:
  Carrots, corn, corn oil, wheat bran and germ.
- Herb sources:
  Alfalfa.

Vitamin P (Bioflavinoids)

- Water soluble.
- Vitamin P is named after paprika, the spice from which it was first isolated. Actually a bioflavinoid complex consisting of rutin, hesperidin and citrin. Found in the pulp of fruits and vegetables.
- Vitamin P aids the functions of vitamin C in keeping collagen (the connective tissue of cells) healthy. It also aids the action of the capillaries in allowing nutrients in and body wastes out. Bio-flavinoids are called the capillary permeability factor. It controls the size of the tiny holes in the capillaries, keeping them large enough to allow nutrients through, but too small for the movement of viruses (which might cause disease) or blood cells (which could lead to local haemorrhage).
- Assists by:
  - working synergistically with vitamin C;
  - strengthens capillary walls;
  - protects against arterial degeneration;
  - builds resistance to disease.
- Herb sources:
  Dandelion, Cayenne, **Red clover, Rose hips.**

Vitamin U

- Many people do not recognise that this vitamin exists. Very little is known about vitamin U.
- Natural sources:
  Grasses.
- Herb sources:
  Alfalfa.

PABA (Para-amino-benzoic Acid)

- Water soluble.
- Part of the B complex family. It is actually a vitamin within a vitamin since it is one of the basic parts of folic acid. It helps with production of folic acid in the intestines. If conditions are right PABA can be synthesised in the intestines.
- It aids in the metabolism of protein, and helps in the assimilation of pantothenic acid.
- PABA is antagonistic to sulfa (synthetic antimicrobials) drugs. Sulfa drugs combine with the same things as PABA so whichever one is in the greater quantity crowds the other out. PABA can make sulfa drugs ineffective and sulfa drugs can cause a PABA deficiency as well as deficiencies of folic acid and pantothenic acid.
- Natural sources:
  Bran, wheat germ.
- Herb sources:
  Alfalfa, Dandelion, Hawthorn, Hops, Kelp, **Red clover**.

The plants listed above are not the only ones on the planet that are sources of vitamins, but the ones listed are common and should be recognised as those found growing in abundance in natural conditions in pastures or country lanes.

It must be noted from sources listed that the dandelion is a very useful herb, as are red clover, and hawthorn. Hops are also listed, as in the past 'brewers grains' were collected from beer makers and fed in small quantities.

Horses will often try to pluck leaves from hawthorn bushes, listed throughout the suggested sources.

It is also interesting to note that bran and linseed are amongst sources of nutrients; horses love a bran mash, especially if it contains linseed. One mash a week is not going to be detrimental.

Kelp is also mentioned, fertilisation using seaweed is a useful source.

Ginger is one of the ingredients of 'old' additives.

Minerals and their herb sources

Minerals constitute a collection of ingredients required by the body for its basic life maintenance processes.

They have a number of functions:

- as catalysts;
- to activate vitamins;
- to become structural components.

All plants extract minerals from soil. Free-ranging animal species will graze the palatable herbage and during the digestive process the body systems extract the required minerals from the broken-down plant matter. Herbs have a high mineral content, adding yet another resource to their obvious dietary attributes.

Minerals tend to be incorporated within the animal's structural architecture. For example, calcium and phosphorus are major components of bone and without them it forms incorrectly, cannot repair efficiently and cannot maintain the required structural design. However, too much of one mineral, or too little of another, can result in a deficiency or incorrect balance between the numerous ingredients necessary for the body to be able to use its calcium/phosphate intake. This is just as hazardous as a lack of either calcium or phosphorus.

Minerals are not manufactured by the body and must be sourced from dietary intake. If the intake is insufficient for the body's requirements, minerals, already involved in a functional role, will be withdrawn for redeployment in another capacity deemed by the body to be of greater importance.

Certain energy processes (for example, muscle activity) require a constant supply of calcium and an inadequacy may well occur during strenuous work. Should this situation arise and not be rectified from food intake, calcium will be removed from bone structures and recycled for use in muscle work, this situation leading to obvious and severe repercussions.

The situation gets more complex once it is realised that for every process of metabolic activity and interaction, a specific vitamin is also required. A shortage, no matter where, in the mineral/vitamin chain will result in functional inefficiency followed by deficiency disease.

Minerals are more complicated than vitamins because they cannot be used by the body in their natural form – they need to be *chelated*. The body must first dissolve the mineral substance and then bind it to a protein molecule. Only then will the blood stream accept the product. Minerals not chelated are excreted; and if a mineral is not accepted, the vitamins it should activate or work with, will in turn become unusable.

In all species, but particularly in the equine athlete, calcium and phosphorus need to be considered as one. They also need an intimate relationship with the 'sunshine' vitamin (D) but unfortunately this is disregarded far too often. Purveyors of additives or feed distributors do not often speak of vitamin D when discussing your horse's requirements.

Calcium and phosphorus contribute the major part of the mineral content of bone. Both are required for efficient muscle activity, and they are also involved in nearly every metabolic function of the body. Vitamin D enhances the correct absorption, retention, mobilisation and deposition of both minerals. Loss of bone density leading to spontaneous fractures has been described by many authors including Krook and Lowe (1964), and confirmed by Cunha (1990).

Calcium is present in chalk, limestone and marble. When fed as an additive it is found in the form of a compound limestone (calcium carbonate), calcium fluoride or calcium sulphate. Phosphorus is highly reactive, and unlike calcium, it does not occur freely in a simple natural form. It is found combined with oxygen as phosphate. Phosphorus is a major component of all cells both in animals and in plants.

Unfortunately, the levels of both minerals are highly variable in all feed. There are many factors to consider: species, maturity, soil content, soil pH, the underground rock strata, climatic conditions, the seed and leaf content, the age of the feed and the harvesting methods all contribute to the concentration levels. One type of food may be high in phosphorus but low in calcium (for example bran), but this can be balanced by introducing a high calcium/low phosphorus ingredient.

The turnip has a 2:1 calcium:phosphorus ratio, so the humble mangold was in fact a source.

Just as with plant-derived vitamin sources all essential minerals can be sourced from the herbage eaten.

Essential minerals

Calcium (Ca)

- Alkaline earth metal.
- Aids in metabolism and is essential to the muscles.
- Must have sufficient vitamin D.
- Calcium loss is retarded by exercise.
- Emotional stress can flush calcium out of the system at a high rate.
- Positive effects:
  - nerve function – impulse transmission;
  - nerve stress;
  - strong bones and teeth;
  - works with magnesium for cardiovascular health;
  - helps regulate the heart beat;
  - helps proper blood clotting;
  - muscle contractions;
  - iron metabolism;
  - helps vitamin C functions.
- Signs of deficiency:
  - poor growth;
  - fragile bones;
  - muscle cramps;
  - weak muscles.
- Natural sources:
  Green vegetables.
- Herb sources:
  Alfalfa, Aloe, Comfrey, Dandelion, Fennel, Garlic, Ginger, Ginseng, **Parsley, Red clover, Red raspberry, Rose hips, Rosemary, Sage.**

Copper (Cu), Molybdenum (Mo)

- Copper and molybdenum interact. Their joint role is not clearly understood, particularly that of molybdenum, but they perform important biochemical as well as nutritional functions.
- Positive effects:
  - play an important role in immunity;
  - are involved in central nervous system functions;
  - assist and are essential for iron activity;
  - assist in collagen metabolism;
  - involved in health of coat;
  - involved in fat metabolism.
- Natural sources:
  Whole grains, leafy green vegetables.
- Herb sources:
  Chickweed, Comfrey, Dandelion, Garlic, Juniper, Kelp, **Peppermint, Red** clover.

Fluorine (F)

- A highly toxic mineral but which appears to be essential in most species. It came to prominence in 1979 when Mandel reported a reduction in dental caries in children if the water supply contained fluoride.

● Contamination by industrial pollution can raise the amount of fluorine in herbage to
  toxic levels.
● Horses affected by excess fluorine may exhibit a dry, rough coat, tight skin, excessive
  tooth wear, poor mastication and chronic pain in all four feet.

Iron (Fe)

● The necessity for iron, like salt, has been recognised since time immemorial.
● Iron is a component of every living organism. It is absorbed throughout the gastroin-
  testinal tract.
● The amount absorbed has been shown to be dependent not only on the source but
  also upon:
   ● the health of the animal;
   ● its age;
   ● the balance of the partnership minerals required by iron to function usefully;
   ● the state of the animal's intestinal tract;
   ● efficient function within the intestinal tract, in particular its pH state.
● Iron is lost in faeces, urine and heavy sweating after exertion.
● Positive effects:
   ● oxygen transport;
   ● activation of oxygen;
   ● functional activities of all cells;
   ● binds to proteins for complex metabolic functions;
   ● assists in immunity;
   ● assists in auto-immune activity;
   ● is involved in *all* body activities.
● Natural sources:
  Whole grain cereals, oatmeal.
● Herb sources:
  Alfalfa, Comfrey, Dandelion, Garlic, Ginger, Hawthorn, Hops, Kelp, Papaya,
  Parsley, Rosemary, Peppermint, Red clover.

Iodine (I)

● Almost all of the trace mineral iodine goes to the thyroid gland to manufacture
  thyroxin.
● Thyroxin is a hormone which affects growth and metabolism.
● Large areas of the planet are *iodine deficient.*
● Positive effects:
   ● The only known effects are associated with the thyroid. Normal growth.
● Sources:
   ● mineral-rich drinking water;
   ● herbage uptake is entirely dependent upon soil conditions;
   ● fertilising the land with seaweed has been shown to improve herbage content.

Manganese (Mn)

● Manganese is a trace material which is needed for normal bone growth and structure.
  It is a catalyst for vitamins B and C. It helps with the proper use of vitamin E.
● It is important to reproduction because it aids in the manufacture of sex hormones
  and lactation.
● Manganese also helps in the formation of thyroxin and in vitamin and carbohydrate
  metabolism.

- Positive effects:
  - skeletal growth;
  - muscle reflexes and co-ordination;
  - important for normal central nervous system;
  - helps eliminate fatigue.
- Natural sources:
  Green leafy vegetables, whole grains.
- Herb sources:
  Chickweed, Garlic, Hops.

Magnesium (Mg)

- Alkaline earth metal.
- Found in compound forms – magnesite, dolomite, etc. It is necessary for the metabolism of calcium, vitamin C, phosphorus, sodium and potassium. Vitamin B_6 helps in the utilisation of magnesium.
- It is used by the body to spark energy (see also *Phosphorus*). Magnesium is lost in urine and faeces.
- Positive effects:
  - helps nerve functions;
  - helps muscle functions;
  - assists blood bearing of oxygen and carbon dioxide;
  - necessary for strong teeth;
  - sparks energy release in body;
  - helps bone growth;
  - prevents calcium deposits;
  - helps mineral metabolism;
  - helps acid/alkaline balance;
  - aids carbohydrate metabolism;
  - helps turn blood sugar to energy.

N.B.: The soil content of magnesium is decreased following heavy dressing with nitrogen and/or potassium.

- Natural sources:
  Fresh green vegetables, wheat germ.
- Herb sources:
  Alfalfa, Dandelion, Ginger, Hops, Red clover, Rosemary, Kelp.

Phosphorus (P)

- Symbolised as a compound (P), e.g. phosphorus and oxygen.
- Stored and used structurally in the bones and teeth.
- Phosphorus is abundant in the body, being present in every cell.
- It is thought that phosphorus plays a role in all the chemical reactions of the body. The form of phosphorus present in the cells and body fluids is called ATP (adenosine triphosphate). ATP is a substance which controls the energy release of the body.
- Magnesium sparks energy and phosphorus controls it. Without magnesium the body would not have any energy and without phosphorus controlling the energy, it would burn itself out.
- Phosphorus is essential to nerve functions, especially those of nerve impulse.
- The brain is largely made up of fats that have been chemically combined with phosphorus.

- Positive effects:
  - normal healthy bones, teeth and gums;
  - cell metabolism;
  - important to nerve function;
  - helps nerve impulse;
  - normal kidney function;
  - necessary for niacin (vitamin B_3) assimilation;
  - proper sugar metabolism;
  - assimilation of proteins;
  - helps convert nutrients to energy.
- Natural sources:
  Whole grains.
- Herb sources
  Alfalfa, Comfrey, Dandelion, Garlic, Ginger, **Hawthorn, Parsley, Raspberry, Rosemary.**

Potassium (K)

- An electrolyte.
- It is not found free in nature and, like phosphorus, is found in combined forms.
- Potassium is sometimes referred to as *potash*. Carbonate of potash is the result of burning organic material and placing the residue in pots to allow it to cool and dry.
- Works with sodium to balance the body fluids, to keep the acid/alkaline balance of those fluids and to regulate the heart beat.
- Potassium is necessary to move substances (nutrients, wastes, etc.) through the cell walls. The body uses what has been called a sodium potassium pump. Potassium works inside the cell walls and sodium works just outside the cell walls. Potassium and sodium are called electrolytes because they carry an electrical charge. It is this electrical charge that 'goes off' and allows the two electrolytes to pump the needed substances in and out of the cells.
- More potassium is needed by the body during any type of stress.
- Positive effects:
  - balances body fluids;
  - acid/alkaline balance of fluids;
  - helps transport oxygen to the brain;
  - helps convert glucose into glycogen;
  - balances sodium;
  - helps the body to grow normally.
- Natural sources:
  Carrots, whole grains.
- Herb sources:
  Alfalfa, Aloe, Dandelion, Echinacea, Garlic, Ginger, **Fennel, Parsley, Raspberry, Rose hips.**

Sodium (Na), Chlorine (Cl), Common salt (NaCl)

- An electrolyte.
- The value of common salt has probably been appreciated since prehistoric times and it has always been a valuable trade commodity. The harvesting of salt from the sea constituted an important industry in many offshore islands until the 1960s when land-excavated salt replaced pure sea salt to a great extent, despite the fact that the latter contains valuable sea-based nutrients.
- Horses sweat more than any other species. They lose salt when sweating as their sweat contains 0.7% salt.

- Once again there is a complication: potassium (K) balances the salt levels and too much potassium results in a salt deficiency. Conversely too much salt will aggravate potassium levels.
- Positive effects:
  - regulation of the balance of body fluids;
  - assists in maintaining heart function;
  - assists in the transmission of nerve impulses;
  - sodium, together with potassium, regulates the acid–base balance.
- Natural sources:
  Rock salt. Allow *free* access. The salt need *not* be mineralised and is usually better accepted as a lump of rock salt.
- Herb sources:
  All herbs contain small amounts of salt but supplementation is needed for animals whose work causes excessive sweating. It is essential to understand that excess sodium chloride (salt) and potassium will *not be stored* for future needs; it will be excreted. As the regulation of body fluids is of the *utmost importance* and is *continually* adjusted, a salt excess over and above the *immediate* requirements of the body will be just as detrimental as a deficiency. It is *vital* to *replace* the lost electrolytes before the fluid balance of the body is seriously disturbed and the animal becomes *dehydrated*, with all the dangerous consequences of that situation.

Sulphur (S)

- Organic sulphur is necessary for all basic body metabolisms.
- Works with the B complex vitamins and is contained in vitamin B_1 *(thiamine)*, vitamin B_5 *(pantothenic acid)* and vitamin H *(biotin)*.
- Sulphur is found in all body proteins; in fact, it is considered a key ingredient in protein, aiding it in all its functions.
- It is lost in urine.
- Positive effects:
  - helps in production of collagen, building of tissue, body repair and maintenance;
  - helps antibody production;
  - helps fight bacterial infections;
  - aids liver in bile secretion;
  - the liver has many enzymes containing sulphur;
  - aids carbohydrate metabolism;
  - attaches with pollutants so they can be removed;
  - incorporated in polypeptide chains;
  - aids carrying of oxygen in blood;
  - helps to maintain oxygen balance necessary for proper brain functions;
  - contained in insulin, adrenalin and thyroxin.
- Natural sources:
  Wheat germ.
- Herb sources:
  Alfalfa, Comfrey, Dandelion, Echinacea, **Fennel,** Kelp, **Parsley, Peppermint, Thyme.**

N.B.: Sulphur requirements are very low. *Flowers of sulphur powder*, fed to horses *can be poisonous* (toxic).

Selenium (Se)

- The need for and feeding of selenium is a serious issue in equine nutrition. Deficiency causes severe muscle disease. For example foals who have been carried by a mare with a selenium deficiency can hardly stand at birth. Older horses have presented with bilateral wastage of specific muscle groups: triceps, quadriceps femoris and the masseter (jaw) muscles. The heart muscle can also be affected.

- *Excess selenium is toxic (poisonous) to the extent that death can result.*
- Interestingly, certain sources of protein, notably *linseed*, achieve a protection against the toxicity of selenium.
- Once again the search for a sensible feed regime leads us back to old methods. At one time a *linseed mash* once, or sometimes twice a week, was a part of a stable routine. The 'feeders' had no scientific backing for their actions but they must have had a reason which must have been improved equine health and performance.
- Positive effects:
  - helps clean cell membranes;
  - works with vitamin E.
- Natural sources:
  Bran.
- Herb sources:
  Garlic, Red clover.

Zinc (Zn)

- Throughout the ancient world zinc is reported as being used as an ointment to cure skin conditions.
- As with iodine, there appear to be large areas on the planet which are zinc deficient.
- Copper needs zinc and zinc needs copper for any process within the body. It is lost in sweat and faeces.
- Positive effects:
  - bound to other elements, zinc assists in:
  - immunity;
  - wound healing;
  - growth;
  - behavioural patterns;
  - genetic translation and transcription;
  - microbial growth;
  - fat metabolism;
  - protection of cell membranes;
  - water balance acting with sodium pumps.
- Natural sources:
  Wheat germ, bran, green leafy vegetables.
- Herb sources:
  Comfrey, Hawthorn, Hops, Kelp.

Conclusion

As with vitamins, it is possible that the full complement of the planet's minerals are as yet undiscovered. The following *must* be present in minute quantities for health but are known to be toxic if consumed in any quantity over a long period:

Aluminium (Al), arsenic (As), cadmium (Cd), lead (Pb), mercury (Hg).

Boron (B), lithium (Li), silicon (Si), and vanadium (V) come under the heading of 'newly discovered' trace elements. To a large extent their role is not fully understood but a total lack of any or all results in deficiency conditions.

It is difficult to portray the complexity of the interaction of every requirement of the living body. It might help to visualise an orchestra and think of the pages of the score, covered with (to the non-musical) endless hieroglyphics. Each means something to every member of the orchestra, but each part of the score relates to the interaction of different musicians, for the notes on those pages represent special functions, each individual has a part to play to complete the whole. However, without instruments the players cannot fulfill their functions, each member of the orchestra must play his or her own role in order to produce a perfect rendering of the piece. The challenges created by different circumstances 'conduct' the way the body must respond – each system is a player, each player needs a complex instrument (think of the number of keys in a piano) with which he or she responds to those demands and all the players must harmonise for the final result – sometimes this will be perfect and sometimes not.

Of the herbal sources listed above as being providers of the necessary vitamins and minerals it is clear that alfalfa (lucerne) is a very nutritious plant. The plant originated in Asia and was taken by merchants to Greece and from there began the Roman usage. 'The Romans were well acquainted with its properties as a forage plant, particularly for horses,' wrote Henry Stephens, FRSE, in 1851.

The plant is described in most comprehensive herbals, particularly those of European origin. *Modern Practical Farriery* published in 1881 (Mackenzie) and *The Book of the Farm* published in 1851 (Stephens), both devote large sections to alfalfa. The crop is said to increase yield annually, reaching maturity in three years. Both authors stress the necessity for a good dressing of 'old yard manure'. Sprangle, in his 1775 paper *The Improved Culture of Lucerne (Alfalfa)*, describes 81 species – I wonder how many are available today?

When discussing hay, the publications mentioned above stressed that 'upland meadow' eight months old was best. Much emphasis is placed on the time of cutting, the number of 'forage' plants required, the time allowed for wilting and the care which must be exercised to avoid excessive seed or leaf loss.

I rather fear modern methods do not allow for such considerations and unfortunately this is a difficult problem to overcome if you are trying to feed a yard full of horses. As a trainer said in despair, 'I simply cannot feed as my father and grandfather did – I cannot get the stuff they used'.

For the single horse owner a 'patch' of alfalfa is quite easy to install, but remember to feed it well, preferably with seaweed.

Cycles of health

When considering athletic activity and the cycles, or seasonal requirements for health, mentioned earlier, it should be remembered that:

1 Many of the components required by the body's 'factories' are not stored for future demand. The body has no ability to plan for the future, and therefore no reason to store surplus for an unpredictable possible demand.

2 The components required for extra or excessive activity can be increased (i.e. storage levels raised) in response to increased exercise demands, so while there is a fine line between too much and too little, if the demands are a *constant* the body will adapt its process of manufacture to meet them, but it will expect a constant balanced demand level. Thus if you are training for a three-mile gallop with the horse expected to carry twelve stone, its ability to perform adequately for the demands imposed by this are unrealistic if it has only been carrying 8 lbs and walking five miles a day!

3 The availability of replacement components for those used during activity is an essential post-activity requirement for adequate recovery. If there is no access to the essential components, the body will borrow/extract from its own tissues the materials required for repair/restoration/replenishment following exertion. This will 'weaken' and render less efficient the structures from which components have been 'borrowed'.

Supplements

Supplementation is poorly understood, and there is a dearth of *proven* experimental information on the absolute levels of minerals required for horses. Maintenance levels are *suggested* but even the requirements of human athletes are constantly adjusted with the discovery of 'new' minerals and vitamins.

One thing is certain – the amounts required are remarkably small.

- Over supplementation is toxic.
- Free choice supplementation is the best approach.
- Supplementation should not be necessary if the quality of herbage contains adequate minerals/vitamins.

I once attended a lecture on feeding for endurance competition horses. The lecturer described his paddocks, the way he made hay and the oats and maize he grew. His horses were only fed his own forage, they looked magnificent, the pastures were old untouched meadows which he proudly pointed out contained 74 species of plants! (See Table 5.1.)

Subsequently, I discovered the pasture was on a seam of a rare soil, known to be mineral rich with the structure described as a green sand belt. Green sand seams appear in various areas and are similar to diatomaceous earth, a highly nutritious source of minerals originating from the pulverised remains of primitive life. Lucky owner, lucky horses.

The storage of forage, no matter what type, is *very* important. Most minerals and vitamins are unstable and are adversely affected by changes in temperature, humidity, packaging, compression or an over-dry atmosphere. The makers of haylage try to prevent nutritional losses by packaging grass forage in a vacuum, but the minute the seal of the vacuum pack is broken the contents begin to oxidise and therefore change. Be careful how and where you store. If the container says 'reseal', then you must reseal, and if there is a 'use by' date the product will be of no benefit and may even do harm if used after that date. Put yourself in your horse's place – you don't eat outdated produce, so why should your horse?

A note of caution: herbs affect body metabolism. They can interact adversely with chemicals i.e.: orthodox drugs, if chemical medication is being administered. *They may also increase threshold levels of body substances which 'enhance performance' above those established as normal.*

The prohibited substance list for horses is extensive and lays down parameters for what are known as *prohibited substance levels*. These are established and refer to any agents which influence:

- the central nervous system;
- the autonomic nervous system;
- the cardiovascular system;
- the gastro-intestinal function;
- the immune system and its response.

Table 5.1 The 74 species identified in old meadows. There is no record of the 20 acres ever having been ploughed.

Scientific name	Common name	Scientific name	Common name
Arrhenatherum elatius	False oat-grass	*Prunella vulgaris*	Selfheal
Poa pratensis	Smooth meadow grass	*Cirsium vulgare*	Spear thistle
Festuca ovina	Sheep's fescue	*Plantago media*	Hoary plantain
Helianthemum nummularium	Common rock-rose	*Centaurea nigra*	Black knapweed
Filipendula vulgaris	Dropwort	*Carex flacca*	Carnation sedge
Plantago lanceolata	Ribwort plantain	*Thymus praecox*	Wild thyme
Dactylis glomerata	Cock's-foot	*Achillea millifolium*	Yarrow
Pimpinella saxifraga	Burnet saxifrage	*Carduus nutans*	Musk thistle
Urtica dioica	Common nettle	*Briza media*	Quaking grass
Medicago lapolina	Black medick	*Reseda lutea*	Wild mignonette
Galium verum	Lady's bedstraw	*Ranunculus repens*	Creeping buttercup
Trisetum flavescens	Golden oat grass	*Silene vulgaris*	Bladder campion
Phleum pratense	Timothy grass	*Myosotis arvensis*	Field forget-me-not
Holcus lanatus	Yorkshire fog	*Potentilla reptans*	Creeping cinquefoil
Crepis capillaris	Smooth hawk's-beard	*Galium mollugo*	Hedge bedstraw
Campanula glomerata	Clustered bellflower	*Vicia cracca*	Tufted vetch
Bromus erectus	Upright broom	*Fragaria vesca*	Wild strawberry
Trifolium pratense	Red clover	*Brachypodium pinnatum*	Tor grass
Campanula rotundifolia	Harebell	*Plantago major*	Great plantain
Agrostis stolonifera	Creeping bent-grass	*Pastinaca sativa*	Wild parsnip
Centaurea scabiosa	Greater knapweed	*Anacamptis pyramidalis*	Pyramidal orchid
Sanguisorba minor	Salad burnet	*Succisa pratensis*	Devil's-bit scabious
Primula veris	Cowslip	*Scabiosa columbaria*	Greater knapweed
Tragopogon pratensis	Goat's-beard	*Polygala calcarea*	Chalk milkwort
Taraxacum officinale	Dandelion	*Gentianella amarella*	Autumn gentian
Cirsium acaulon	Dwarf thistle	*Asperula cynanchia*	Squinancywort
Veronica chamaedrys	Germander speedwell	*Picris hieracioides*	Bristly ox-tongue
Arenaria serpyllifolia	Thyme-leaved sandwort	*Stachys officinalis*	Betony
Cerastium fontanum	Common mouse-ear	*Rumex acetosa*	Common sorrel
Senecio vulgaris	Groundsel	*Sambucus nigra*	Elder
Sonchus asper	Pricky sow-thistle	*Koeleria macrantha*	Crested hair-grass
Linum catharticum	Fairy flax	*Ligustrum vulgare*	Wild privet
Leontodon hispidus	Rough hawkbit	*Rhamnus catharticum*	Alder buckthorn
Lotus corniculatus	Common bird's-foot trefoil	*Betula pendula*	Silver birch
Senecio jacobaea	Common ragwort	*Trifolium repens*	White clover
Leucanthemum vulgare	Ox-eye daisy	*Viola hirta*	Hairy violet
Knautia arvensis	Field scabious	*Crataegus monogyna*	Hawthorn

Herbs act as:

- antibiotics;
- antihistamines;
- anti-malarial and anti-parasitic agents;
- anti-pyretic, analgesic and anti-inflammatory substances;
- diuretics;
- local anaesthetics;
- muscle relaxants;
- respiratory stimulants.

They influence:

- sex hormones;
- endocrine secretions;
- substances affecting blood coagulation;
- cytotoxic substances.

It is important to realise that 'going alternative' rather than 'using orthodox' does *not* mean your horse will automatically 'test negative'. However, provided your horse has been allowed a 'balanced' intake rather than an 'excess' all will be well.

Summary

The previous pages have suggested the benefits of allowing the horse to select naturally from fresh organic sources. Common herbs are named in order to demonstrate the micronutrients (vitamins) and minerals which can be sourced from various types of plant, always provided those plants were grown in soil containing the nutrients the plants require and that the ground had not been exhausted by intensive agriculture or chemical manipulation. It is *not* a complete list.

All the information included is intended to promote health. It is for *nutritive* herbal use, not *curative* herbal use. Those who wish to 'treat' ill health or injury must seek veterinary advice as *no treatment* will be effective unless the *correct diagnosis* is obtained first. Once a diagnosis has been made, a study of the medicinal properties of herbs is necessary for it is unwise to 'doctor' at random.

Juliette de Bairacli Levy (1991) quotes Louis Bromfield who, in his book *Pleasant Valley*, writes that any person in charge of land or animals 'has to know more things than a person in any other profession; he or she has to be a biologist, a veterinary, a mechanic, a botanist, a horticulturist, a stockman and many other things'. This is certainly true for the maintenance of health, you cannot cook successfully without the correct balance of ingredients, neither can you build your horse without balance in all aspects of care.

Further reading

Abrams, J.T. In *Handbook Series in Nutrition and Food*, Section E: Nutritional Disorders, (M. Recheigl, Ed.), CRC Press, Florida

de Bairacli Levy, J. *Herbal Handbook for Farm and Stable*, revised edn, Faber and Faber, London, 1991

Culpeper, N. *Culpeper's Complete Herbal*, (originally pubd 1653), Wordsworth Editions Ltd, Ware, Herts, 1995

Gutmanis, J. *Kahuna La'au Lapa'au – Hawaiian Herbal Medicine*, Island Heritage, Hawaii, 1987

Haas, E. M. *Staying Healthy With the Seasons*, Celestial Arts, Berkeley, CA, 2004

Hills, L.D. *Russian Comfrey*, Faber & Faber, London, 1953

Lust, J. *The Herb Book*, Bantam Books, Transworld, London, 1990

Miles, W.J. *Modern Practical Farriery*, William Mackenzie, London, 1881

Mervyn, L. *The Dictionary of Vitamins*, Thorsons, London, 1984

Malstrom, S. *Own Your Own Body*, Woodland, London, 1988

Stephens, H. *The Book of the Farm*, Vols I & II, Blackwood, London, 1881

Stuart, M. (Ed.), *The Encyclopedia of Herbs*, Macdonald & Co., London, 1979

Vogel, H.C.A. *The Nature Doctor*, Mainstream, Edinburgh, 1990

Part II

Therapies

6

Homoeopathy

To the discerning reader it is clear that herbalism, homoeopathy, acupuncture or acupressure require in-depth study in order to practise any one of them safely and effectively. There is no instant learning curve and it is beyond the scope of this book to teach all the detail of the subjects. The aim is to expose readers to the complexities of age-old methods concerned with health. All the subjects were originally learnt in the traditional way by an apprenticeship which lasted for years under a master.

There is some confusion about the differences between herbal medicine and homoeopathic medicine, particularly as both derive their basic ingredients from natural resources. The main difference can be understood when it is appreciated that in homoeopathy there is no standard remedy for a known condition. Each individual case should be separately assessed and a specific remedy prescribed. The remedies will vary and those chosen should be related to the whole. This must take into account the environment, personality and character of the patient, as well as the symptoms experienced. Patients who turn to homoeopathic medicine find they are healthier and the reports from owners using homoeopathic vets give similar results.

Current medical thinking is that it is the symptoms of a condition which need to be treated, homoeopathy considers that the symptoms are the reactive efforts or responses of the body's defence systems to an invasion and these symptoms need to be stimulated rather than suppressed. The principal of *similia similibus curentur*, let like be treated by like, is employed in order to achieve this.

Hippocrates, the Greek physician from the fifth century BC, recognised this principle, as did the Swiss alchemist, Paracelsus, in the sixteenth century, but it was left to Dr Samuel Hahnemann, born in Saxony in 1755, to 'rediscover' the idea. It was he who evolved the name homoeopathy from the Greek language – 'homoios' for like and 'pathos' for suffering. Hahnemann was a gifted man, he spoke nine languages, was a chemist and then became a doctor of medicine, and it was while translating the *Materia Medica* by Professor Cullen of Edinburgh that he began to experiment upon himself. When he took quinine, or as it was then known Cinchona bark, a known remedy for malaria, he found that he developed symptoms indistinguishable from those of malaria itself. A little later, in 1796, Dr Edward Jenner used the secretions from cows with cowpox to vaccinate people and prevent them from contracting smallpox.

Hahnemann continued to experiment by giving single remedies to volunteers. Between 1779 and 1832 his research contributed 112 papers. Substantial proof was required by the apothecaries of the day whose medical practices included bleeding, cupping and the use of toxic elements such as arsenic, repeatedly prescribed in ever larger quantities if a cure was not effected. Proof of Hahnemann's ability to cure by his methods came in 1821 when the battle of Leipzig ended with a typhoid epidemic. Hahnemann treated 180 cases and only one patient died. In 1831 of the 154 cases of cholera he treated, only 6 died, while of the 1500 treated by the then 'orthodox' methods 821 died. The principles handed down from Hahnemann form the basis of practising homoeopaths of today.

Arguments continue as to the validity of homoeopathic remedies, due in the main to the dilution of the initial component. Hahnemann dosed his healthy volunteers with various substances and continued until they produced symptoms resembling a known illness. Once it was established that a particular substance had evoked a symptom or symptoms it was subjected to dynamisation, with one drop of the mother tincture (substance) being diluted with 99 drops of alcohol and the mixture shaken vigorously. This shaking (succussion) is essential for the preparation of remedies and the process is repeated until the required dilution (potency) is achieved. Hahnemann had 'proved' 99 mother tinctures before his death in 1843.

Today the preparation of homoeopathic remedies still uses the processes of dynamisation and succussion to achieve the required potency, exactly as described by Hahnemann, despite the fact that it has been scientifically proven that after the ninth dynamisation not a single molecule of the original substance remains. Critics claim the effects are placebo. If this is so, why do homoeopathic remedies prove so beneficial in animal therapy?

Questions and theories on how homoeopathic remedies work abound:

- Can such an infinitesimal dose permeate or chemically influence the cell membrane?
- Can disorientated receptors recognise the energy imprint of the original substance and use it to restabilise?
- Does the remedy set up vibratory interactions disturbed by toxic reactions?

Whatever the reason, homoeopathy undoubtedly has a role both in prevention and cure.

As with any extrinsic interference, it is unwise just to buy a remedy and 'try it'. Homoeopathy evolved after much experimentation by a medical man who was also a chemist. He understood, even though limited by eighteenth-century knowledge, the problems of health and the signs and symptoms of disease. The science he recognised is practised successfully by people who have been trained at specialist schools, many of whom have previously qualified as doctors or vets.

Homoeopathy, like Chinese medicine, requires considerably more observation than orthodox medicine so you can help your homoeopathic vet by carrying out constant surveillance of your animal/s. When any therapy is given it is both helpful and advisable to note down the behaviour of your horse and its reactions over a period of time.

Homoeopathic first aid

If you, the owner, or groom have a good relationship with your homoeopathic vet, it is helpful to have a small selection of remedies for first aid. These can be purchased either from the vet or a good homoeopathic pharmacy, such as Ainsworths in London.

The potencies of homoeopathic remedies are indicated by a number. This may be followed by the letter x. For example 6x potency contains 1/1,000,000 part of the total original substance. Those remedies styled 'high' potencies, 200th, 1r, 10r, etc. are those with the most minute amounts of the basic preparation. The most commonly used potency on sale to the general public is 6x; most qualified practitioners dispense from their own pharmacies choosing the potency required following examination and diagnosis.

Suggested first aid kit

In the absence of professional advice, choose the remedy most appropriate for the situation. Do not give the animal several remedies in case one is 'better' than another.

Aconite (aconitum napellus) Common Monkshood

- Uses: relieves pain, sedates temporarily.
- Of the same family as the buttercup. The remedy is obtained from a part of the root system.
- The plant is poisonous to carnivores but less so to herbivores.
- The remedy can be in tablet or liquid format.

Arnica (arnica montana)

- Uses: bruising both superficial and deep. Filling in joints.
- The plant grows in the mountain pastures of central Europe where the soil is calcareous.
- The remedy is obtained from the flowers and rhizomes.
- The remedy can be in the form of tablets, lotion or cream.

Belladonna (atrope bella-donna) Deadly Nightshade

- Uses: pain killer, tissue antispasmodic, anti-asthmatic, all via its effect on the nervous system.
- The plant is poisonous, particularly to species with a highly developed nervous system. It should never be used if the animal is bleeding, as its effects are to increase rather than decrease haemorrhage.
- The remedy is obtained from the leaves and roots.
- The remedy can be taken as a tablet or used as a tincture.

Hypericum (hypericum perforatum) St Johns Wort

- Uses: grazes, broken skin, bruised nerves.
- The remedy is obtained from the tips of the fresh flowers.
- The remedy can be taken in a fluid or as a syrup. A fluid extract or oil can be applied directly to the damaged area.

Witch Hazel (hamamelis virginiana)

- Uses: reduces bleeding by constricting blood vessels.
- Useful for immediate first aid for tendon strain.
- Effective following bruising, particularly in the back.
- The plant grows as a garden shrub in the UK and it is found in the wild state in North America.
- The remedy is obtained from the leaves.
- The remedy is best applied as a tincture or infusion externally over the damaged area.

With experience the basic first aid kit will grow to contain an increased number of remedies.

Many seem to have similar effects. The question is: 'how do I decide which to use?' You must ask yourself questions;

- Aconite and belladonna both relieve pain, but do you need general sedation as well as pain reduction or do you need to ease pain and reduce tension in the tissues after local damage?
- Aconite relieves pain but also sedates.
- Belladonna reduces pain and relieves local spasm.

- If the horse has had an accident and is upset, aconite might be the choice but if the horse has been kicked, belladonna would possibly suit better.

You must try to choose the remedy most appropriate to the symptoms and the individual's needs.

Many of the plants sources used in homoeopathy to aid the body to recover from adverse occurrences are classified as poisonous, that is they are toxic in their natural state. Once the remedy has been extracted and been subjected to the processes associated with achieving the correct potency, and provided the prescribed dose is not exceeded, the effects of the substance are considered to neutralise the adverse effects of the condition for which it has been shown to be pertinent.

Homoeopathy, like herbalism, is effective. It is classified as 'alternative' but this does not mean it is easy to use.

Further reading

de Bairacli Levy, J. *Herbal Handbook for Farm and Stable*, Faber & Faber, London, 1991

Blackie, M.G. *The Challenge of Homoeopathy*, Unwin, London, 1984

Buchman, D.D. *Ancient Healing Secrets*, Ottenheimer, Owings Mills, USA, 1996

Chiej, R. *The Macdonald Encyclopedia of Medicinal Plants*, Macdonald & Co., London, 1984

Livingston, R. *Homoeopathy, Evergreen Medicine*, Asher Press, Poole, UK, 1991

Macleod, G. *The Treatment of Horses by Homoeopathy*, Eastern Press Ltd, London, 1983

Macleod, G. *A Veterinary Materia Medica*, The C.W. Daniel Co. Ltd, Saffron Walden, UK, 1983

Self, H.P. *A Modern Horse Herbal*, Kenilworth Press, Addington, UK, 2001

7 Bach Flower Remedies

No account of homoeopathy would be complete without a mention of the Bach Flower Remedies. Dr Bach was a doctor of medicine who first worked in public health, then studied bacteriology. In the early 1900s, dissatisfied with orthodox medical attitudes he turned to homoeopathy as he, like Hahnemann, was certain that the emotional state of the patient contributed to their health problems.

His training as a bacteriologist led him to examine the intestinal flora of patients in his care. Intestinal flora are bacteria normally present within the intestines, even in health. Bach discovered that chronic conditions changed the normal patterns of these flora and each condition gives rise to its own peculiar archetype of disturbance. Bach isolated seven groups of intestinal flora and from nosodes, using homoeopathic principals, he prepared remedies. A nosode describes material extracted from the product of a disease. The patient is 'dosed' with a minute amount of the product in order to effect a cure.

The use of a preparation extracted from the saliva of dogs with rabies had been used to treat humans suffering from hydrophobia as early as 1833, so the practice was not new. However, the main difference was that after he isolated what are still called the seven bowel (intestinal) nosodes, Bach prescribed the appropriate remedy. This was not done after considering the patient's symptoms (for example, the fever, colic, a cough, pain) but according to the emotional state or temperament of the person. A patient suffering from a stomach ulcer would be treated for worry/anxiety, the remedy used being chosen as appropriate for that patient's mental condition. Orthodox medical practitioners were not convinced despite, at this stage in his career, the scientific background to the work.

In 1930, Bach left London and moved to the country to seek remedies from nature for emotional states. It is said that he became highly mentally and physically sensitive. In a self-described 'negative' state of mind he would set off and wander through unspoilt country until he chanced upon a flower which he felt restored his mental and physical serenity. Between 1930 and 1936, when he died, he had chosen 38 flowers from trees and plants to counteract what he considered were the 38 adverse mental states which man might experience, disease-induced or not. The remedies could, he considered, be used to prevent the onset of physical conditions as the mental state was relieved.

Despite the fact that all Bach's work related to human disease and the intestinal flora of the human gut, the Bach Flower Remedies are used by many people for their animals. Stacey Small, the founder of Holistic Horse, has successfully transposed Bach's ideals producing, following research, a range of essences appropriate for animals and known as the Botanical Animal Flower Essences. Once again we are back to nature-derived components taken from the world of plants.

Horses are undoubtedly temperamental, so it is important for the natural horseman to learn to read their horse, as they will interpret and classify their horse's 'mood' prior to choosing the appropriate remedy.

Rescue Remedy

Many people carry Rescue Remedy, a conglomerate of five of the 38 remedies identified by Bach. Described as a remedy for emergencies it is evolved from:

- clematis to avoid fainting;
- cherry plum to control hysteria;
- impatiens to relax physical and emotional tension;
- rock rose to avoid fear and/or panic reactions;
- star of Bethlehem to alleviate shock.

For the average, horse the suggested dosage is ten drops in the water bucket or four drops on a sugar lump.

The mother tinctures of all the remedies are prepared using the petal tips of the fresh flowers from the appropriate plants. Just as with other complementary therapies, correct selection is the most important factor for success.

The art of prescribing requires an in-depth study of equine mentality and its response to stress. Very little published work is available. If the remedies are as effective as they are claimed to be, misreading a situation would make things worse rather than better.

8 Past-Age Remedies

Remedies for common problems associated with the horse, rather than disease, are described in early writing, usually in texts for farriers, for in the past, the shoeing smith or farrier doubled as the horse doctor. In today's terms, the word blacksmith is often incorrectly used, in the original terminology the blacksmith worked with metal, the farrier shod, had an in-depth knowledge of the equine foot and was the equine podiatrist.

The ingredients for many old remedies, such as arsenic for coughs, and red lead, an ingredient in red blister, used for tendon injuries are no longer available. Some ingredients which are still viable are described, but none should be used without veterinary discussion and agreement.

Many old remedies have been analysed in recent years and the claims attributed verified.

Bread poultice

- Uses: to draw pus, a deeply imbedded thorn or other foreign material from a wound, treat a badly bruised sole.
- Method:
  1 Take a thick slice of white bread, place between two squares of, preferably, absorbent white lint (available from chemists). If no lint is available, two towel squares can be used.
  2 Dip into a pan of boiling water.
  3 When soaked, wring out, and as the pad cools to a tolerable warmth, place over the target area.
  4 Cover and wrap area in cotton wool.
  5 Cover and wrap area in cling film.
  6 Secure with a stable bandage.
  7 Leave overnight.

Bran poultice

- Uses: as for bread poultice.
- Method: as for bread poultice, replacing the slice of bread with a good scoop of bran to create a wedge or depth of at least 5 cm between the two squares of lint or towelling.

Botanical Animal Flower Essences

Based on the flower essences identified by Dr Edward Bach the preparations are ready to use, derived from pure sources, they are useful for owners who do not have either access to or the inclination to gather and prepare the essences as described by Bach.

Comfrey poultice

- Uses: bruises and local filling on body or limbs.
- Method:
  1 Take five or six fresh comfrey leaves.
  2 Place in a shallow container.
  3 Cover with hot (not boiling) water.
  4 When soft (1 to 1^{1}/2 minutes) wrap around target area.
  5 If the leaves can be held in place with a bandage finish as for bread poultice.
  6 If the bruised area is on the body mass, soak the leaves, cover with warm water and leave to soak overnight, strain off the liquor into a jar or bottle. Use to soak the target area, two or three times a day.

Cabbage poultice

- Uses: filled legs.
- Method: as for comfrey poultice.

Sauerkraut – Pickled white cabbage

- Uses: bruised areas, particularly bruised soles.
- Method:
  1 Clean out the foot, pack with the sauerkraut.
  2 Hold in place, either using a plastic wrap or a child's disposable nappy. (The latter are used by many top-flight event grooms to hold poultices in place for foot problems!)
  3 Leave overnight.

Goose grease

- Uses: to encourage hair growth, naturally coloured, rather than white following a skin lesion or break down.
- Method:
  1 Paint a thin covering over a scar, or skin lesion.
  2 Use every second to third day, *do not rub in.*
  3 **N.B.:** If rubbed in hard you will blister the area.

Honey (pure honey)

- The use of honey is a text in its self. Honey for wounds is described in 4000-year-old Egyptian texts.
- Interestingly, current research has shown that honey breaks down to a common disinfectant, hydrogen peroxide.
- Uses: open wounds.
- Method: cover the open area with liquid honey.
- With crushed garlic added, honey was used for coughs.

Linseed

- Uses: said to cleanse the horse.
- Method:
  1 A tea is made, by mixing one pound of linseed with a gallon of water.
  2 The mix should be placed on a stove or in a warm area and left simmering very slowly for 12 hours.
  3 The jelly-like liquid is poured off and half to quarter of a pint mixed into a normal bran mash.
  4 Feed once weekly on the night before the rest day.

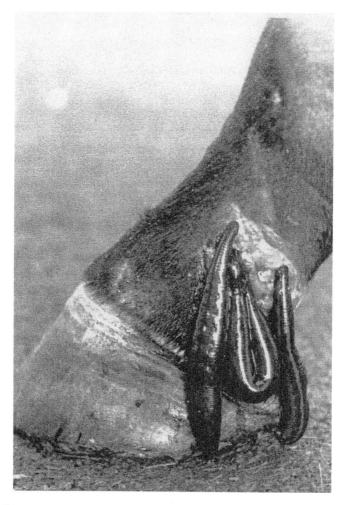

Fig. 8.1 Leeches: useful for stimulating wound healing.

Leeches

- Medicinal leeches have been used for centuries, they are available in the twenty-first century from the leech farm in South Wales (see Fig. 8.1; Useful addresses section, page 234).
- Uses: to stimulate healing in wounds, particularly chronic wounds.
- Method: apply the leeches to the wound, leave until they drop off.
- The leech has a triangular mouth. It lives off blood and excretes heparin within the area of mouth attachment. Heparin reduces the clotting mechanism present in blood ensuring a resumption/increase of local circulatory flow. This enhances healing.
- (The author has used this method with veterinary approval on badly lacerated knees, with great success.)

Nettles

- An old gypsy remedy for laminitis.
- Uses: laminitis, other inflammatory foot problems.

- Method: pick some, preferably young nettles, leave them to wilt for several hours. Offer them to the horse.
- Nettles were also used as a tonic, reasonable as they are now known to be a source of vitamin C and iron.
- **N.B.**: some horses are allergic to nettles.

Sore No More

- A twenty-first-century product, based on a receipt of herbs used for centuries by the American Indians.
- Uses: bruising, filled joints secondary to sprains, muscle damage.
- Method: saturate the target area.

Water
Gypsies and other travellers have always made use of streams with a solid base, standing horses often tied to a tree, for periods of up to an hour 'to cool legs'. Horses enjoy the experience and many trainers stand or walk their horse in water (Fig. 8.2).

Sea water
For those near the sea, almost nothing beats wading, particularly following minor leg problems. The sand stimulates balance receptors in the feet and because of the saline nature of the water osmosis occurs, excess fluids in the limb are drawn out through the porous skin.

Rolling
Horses should be encouraged to roll after ridden exercise, this allows their backs to self adjust. There is no debate regarding the fact that horses can suffer from back ache, but they *do not commonly*, unlike man and the dog, slip discs or suffer from gross inter-vertebral malalignment.

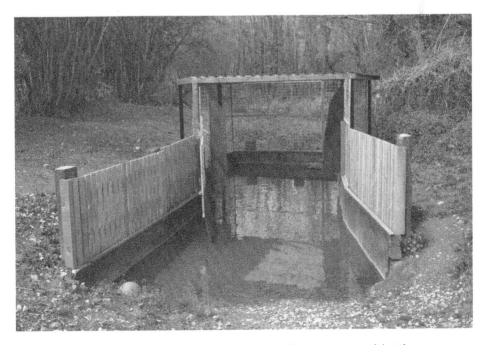

Fig. 8.2 A running stream has been 'captured', horses stand in the pen to cool their legs.

Allowing a horse to roll enables the animal to influence the back because the muscles of the vertebral column are relieved from the necessity to support the weight of the abdominal contents and counteract gravitational pull. These are the two forces the column must resist in the standing position, requiring considerable muscle tension.

Post-exercise rolling *in no way* resembles colic rolling.

Prior to the Second World War all large stables had a rolling area, usually covered in sand. After exercise, horses were led to the area on a lunge line and encouraged to roll. It would be reasonable to suggest this reduced the likelihood of the horse getting down in its box to roll, a situation that often results in the horse getting cast and injuring its back.

The following selection of horse remedies, for amusement only, were taken verbatim in 1968 from originals held in Netherthorpe Grammar School. They were collected by The Rev Gisbourne, Rector of Staveley, Derbyshire, circa 1800.

Epidemical coughs and colds
Take 1 pint best vinegar, boil it then take off scum. Put in a lump of fresh butter or a spoonful of sweet oil. When lukewarm, add it to a new laid egg, mix it well and give to the horse fasting, for three mornings. If the horse has a rattling in his head mix sulphur with fresh butter and with a goose feather put it up the nostril and confine it for half an hour. Ride him about.

To kill worms in horses
Take as much red precipite as will lie on a silver three pence. Make it up with fresh butter into pills, wrap it up in paper silk give it with the horse fasting at least two hours then give scalded bran and warm water or gruel. Then give a gentle purge to work it off three or three and a half hours after. Walk the horse well.

Another remedy to kill worms
Take four ounces of powdered tin and make into a ball with soft soap and give it the horse and the next morning give him a dose of Physick and work it well off and the all will come away.

For a strain or bruise
Take Oil of Thyme 2 pence, Oil of Swallows 2 pence, Oil of worms 2 pence, Oil of Vitriol pennyworth, Oil of Turpentine 2 penny worth, Oil of Spike 2 pence, Spirit of Wine 2 pence,
Mix all. Rub on well it is excellent for a strain.

For a strain in the back
A gang of calves feet stewed with half an ounce of Harts horn shavings, and half an ounce of Isinglass. All mixed. It has been found excellent good.

Greasy heels
Take train oil and whitening, mix it well with a mortar till a fine ointment. Clip off the heels and rub in well, at the same time give Duiretick balls, and it never fails to cure.

9 Health Maintenance and Healing

Texts recording the practice of healing, BC, do not appear anywhere other than in China. In chronological order, Chinese healing, which includes the use of acu stimulation, massage, and the use of herbs, appears to predate other therapies.

Before discarding conventional methods it is sensible to have some knowledge of the age-old methods and to decide if they really are applicable, in a beneficial manner, for your situation. Always consider the fact that by the introduction of any interference, external or internal, a response, even a series of responses, will be initiated in the system or organ you target, and by so doing over-riding, influencing and manipulating the inbuilt reactions and processes with which the body is naturally endowed.

Acu procedures are described in some detail in this text, *not* to teach the subject, but in order to give the reader an idea of the far-reaching investigative procedures practised when using these methods; also to indicate the importance of detailed observation of the body responses not only to an illness, but including lifestyle and the effects of the elements. In this way, diagnosis is based on a very broad approach.

Those practising the trade we call medicine were primarily interested in keeping their patients healthy. This is hardly surprising as they only got paid *if the health of the subject, animal or human, was maintained, but not when they became unwell.*

However hard the natural horseman attempts to maintain his animal's health, from time to time some form of assistance may be necessary. This may be to enhance the health of the subject, or to restore health, following accident, injury or exposure to infection.

The world has changed dramatically, as have the range of accidents and disease, since methods of treatment were first described therefore it must be asked, are methods originating in prehistory still appropriate?

It is worth considering that when massage and acupressure were first recorded as written texts in China, at the time of the Yellow Emperor who invented writing (then charmingly described as 'the script of birds' footprints'), Chinese civilisation had already been in existence for thousands of years. Until this time, 2740 BC, information had been handed down by example and word of mouth. It is not until 722 BC that treatment charts for animals appear. It is interesting to note that the horse is only described with meridians, while the camel, pig and even hens have points illustrated.

A body, no matter what the species, is endowed with its own in-built methods which enable it to attempt to recover following health breakdown. The senior vets often still say, 'leave it to nature'. However, when help is required, the choice of therapy or treatment, when seeking to adopt any one of the alternative methods of health manipulation, is far more difficult than pursuing orthodox/conventional medical methods. It must be understood that none are a DIY substitute. Alternative therapies present a far greater challenge than conventional medicine, there are no fixed formulae, no fixed rules and the goal posts are continuously on the move. *The attitude that alternative therapies are 'easier' and can be prescribed and practised by anyone, could not be further from the truth.*

As explained previously in this text the importance of the ability 'to read' your horse through routine, daily observation was discussed. All 'alternative' therapies require a wider range of detailed information to aid diagnosis than conventional medicine. There are a significant number of points to consider.

Assessment

Listed below are some of the factors to which your horse may react and any abnormal behaviour patterns you might notice. Your observation of all or any reactions will help your alternative therapist in his/her general assessment. Observations and reactions to notice include:

- *Climate:*
  Heat, cold, humidity, rain, thunder, wind, sun.
- *Diet:*
  Barley, oats, bran, nuts, mixes, linseed, sugar beet, haylage, meadow hay, lucerne hay, water.
  Drinks a lot, drinks little, eats up, leaves food, eats earth, licks a lot of salt.
- *Bedding:*
  Reaction to, paper, shavings, straw.
  Eats bedding, digs a central pit.
- *Temperament:*
  Restless, temper flashes, over-sensitive, dull, unco-operative.
- *Reaction to rider or groom:*
  Angry, friendly, moves away, no co-operation.
- *Posture:*
  Leans, sits back on walls.
  Always lying down, never lies down.
  Rolls constantly.
  Rests a leg, points a leg.
- *Sensations:*
  Sweats, easily, in patches, for no reason.
  Itches, paws the ground, crib bites, wind sucks.
  Legs fill. Hind only? Front only?
  Resents girth or roller, cold backed when mounted.
- *Pain:*
  Kicks out for no reason, bucks for no reason, rolls often, bites sides, looks tucked up.
- *Incorrect movement:*
  Disunited, avoids a lead, will not bend on a circle.
  Rests a leg when possible.
  Head shakes, avoids contact with the bit.
- *General health:*
  Spotty coat, dull coat.
  Runny nose, runny eyes.
  Pale lower eyelids.
  Tight skin.
  Dehydrated.
  Sparse thick urine.
  Eats droppings, dry droppings, sloppy droppings.
  Bad breath, quids food.

Pale or black gums, stained teeth.

Poor hoof growth.

- *Never well since:*

Medication, cough, accident, colic, vaccination, anaesthetic, competition, fall, change of diet, change of bedding.

- *General appearance:*

Alert, dull.

Dry coat.

Pale below eyes.

Ringed hoof growth.

Cats hairs under jaw remain despite coat change.

Runny eyes, runny nose, early fatigue when exercised.

Slow cardiovascular recovery after exercise.

10 Acupuncture and Acupressure

In historical records, stimulation of the body by pressure, acupressure, is the first technique described. The tip of a finger, usually that of the referring physician, being the tool used to apply pressure. Following diagnosis, appropriate points were selected and the intensity of pressure was stipulated, this depending on the presumed depth of the point.

As senior members of the Chinese hierarchy became more 'god like', they could not be touched by a commoner, and so pressure was applied by the use of pointed stones, with needle puncture arriving even later.

The exact location of all points was described using anatomical landmarks, so surface anatomy, or the recognition of surface landmarks, was very important. An important consideration when using acupressure on horses, but which is often ignored, is the flexibility of equine skin when compared with that of man, this makes it difficult to be accurate in point location on the horse.

In the West, we tend to think of acupuncture as a single therapy. This is an incorrect concept, as acupuncture is a part of the 'whole' in traditional Chinese medicine; no patient would, for example, undergo surgery without the inclusion of acupuncture. Western medicine is compartmentalised, surgery practised as a single entity, the patient usually finding themselves referred to several other doctors each of whom specialise in a single aspect of their condition, which is often multifactorial.

In the West, you cannot practise medicine without sufficient knowledge of anatomy and disease to enable a diagnosis to be made. In the same way, no one should practise acupuncture unless they understand the basic principles of the philosophy of Chinese traditional medicine, and this includes the making of a diagnosis, mental or physical.

For acupuncture to be successful, no matter which technique is used to influence the *points*, it is essential to understand that due to the interaction of all body systems, triggering one, primary reaction, no matter where it occurs will not be locally confined – the effects will concern and affect the whole body.

It is amazing to learn that over 5000 years ago the physicians considered that each organ interacted with all the other organs, and for good function there had to be balance throughout the whole. This is a concept which appears largely to have diminished in the modern, chemical treatment approach, when the 'side effects' of many therapies seem to be worse than the condition.

The popularity of the use of acupuncture has waxed and waned over time despite the fact that known Chinese treatments date back thousands of years. In the early 1970s, acupuncture was 're-invented' and began to be extensively practised in the West. It is likely that the preceding lack of usage of this therapy stemmed from the fact that the philosophy behind Chinese medicine, requiring the whole and not just the symptoms to be considered, was totally alien to western medical practices, wherein the symptoms were treated and the whole rarely considered. A further consideration needs addressing which may also be a possible reason for continuing scepticism of the efficacy of acu therapies in the West. While Chinese medicine aims to achieve *balance* and prevent sickness, Western medicine treats the after-effects of sickness. It must also be emphasised that there are now large numbers of conditions probably not present, and certainly not diagnosed, some 5000 years ago.

No one can debate the requirement for the body systems to be in balance. Due to the process of evolution, which now includes longevity, an undreamed of, intimate knowledge of the body structures, and an increase in the number of diagnosed conditions, it is reasonable to suggest that Chinese medicine might helpfully be integrated with Western, rather than existing in isolation; particularly as research has demonstrated that the anatomical *points* described in Chinese medicine have been proven to be small areas of lowered electrical resistance on the skin.

In Western medicine, descriptive diagnosis is coupled to long incomprehensible names, often leading to problems becoming exacerbated by fear. The Chinese approach embraces acceptable and therefore 'fear free' concepts because their diagnostic terminology is not alien but rather is related to components of daily living – light, fire, water, sweat, bitter, sweet, spicy. This usage of everyday expressions means people already have experience of the descriptive terms and can relate to similar characteristics in matters of health or illness, be it their own or that of their animals.

The fact that balance is necessary, not only throughout the body but also in life is now beginning to become accepted in the West and for those attempting natural horse care this is an important consideration. Horses are herd animals, the freedom to roam with other horses, even just to see and to communicate with their own kind establishes a more acceptable 'life' balance. Many stable 'vices' arise from boredom, of which solitary confinement is the worst. Think of people jailed, when solitary confinement is considered to be the worst punishment.

Basic principles of traditional Chinese veterinary medicine

Yin and yang

Early Chinese teachings considered that there were principal underlying laws which governed the universe, both physical and metaphysical. One of the accepted principles was that there was a constant interaction between opposites as they endeavoured to achieve balance, this balance requirement is known as *yin* and *yang*.

Yin is considered to have a negative, or passive, quality while *yang* is considered to have an active, or positive, quality. Every organic and inorganic object within the known universe is classified as being either yin or yang. Within the philosophy of Chinese medicine it is considered that any upset of the yin-to-yang balance creates a situation that allows for the onset of disease or for a state of being unwell.

Meridians (connecting energy paths)

Traditional Chinese acupuncture describes twelve *meridians* or paths for energy flow. It is considered that these meridians enable the movement of energy or *ch'i*. The paths are described as routes interlinking all the body organs, not only to each other, but also to the body surface. The meridian network is not as comprehensive for animals as it is for the human subjects.

These descriptions of energy flow could, in the light of increased interest in, and understanding of, the *autonomic nervous system*, be compared to the message interaction between organs and the body surface now known to exist and to be governed by the autonomic section of the general nervous system.

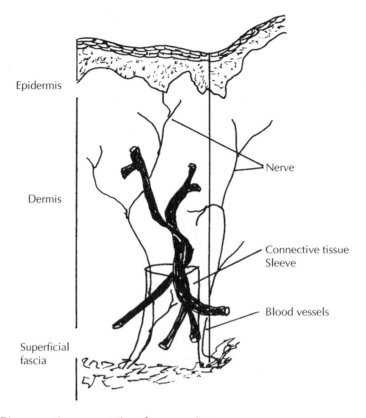

Epidermis

Nerve

Dermis

Connective tissue
Sleeve

Blood vessels

Superficial
fascia

Fig. 10.1 Diagrammatic representation of an acu point.

Points (see Fig. 10.1)

Points are precise locations on the skin's surface which, when stimulated, will achieve a calculated response. Research shows that acu points are well endowed with neural receptors. In addition, the area of the skin lying above each acu point exhibits considerably less resistance to the passage of weak electrical currents than does the surrounding skin. This lowered resistance can be detected by electrical recorders, but skilled operators, able to detect points by touch, describe them as having a slightly differing texture – being found in small depressions – with the local texture feeling softer.

In Chinese texts, precise measurements for identification are given, a known anatomical landmark is selected, then both direction and distance from the feature are given. Many *trigger points* described in massage texts, are located in similar positions to acu points and it is interesting to observe that the described paths of some equine meridians mirror known 'zone lines' of the horse (an area of increased skin tension). These lines also mirror the path of described lymphatic drainage channels (see Fig. 10.2).

The *ch'i*, or energy (which may be yin or yang), flows in a specific pattern within the meridian network. The identified points for organ stimulation are located on the *paths* of these meridians.

The body organs, their functions and reactions are classified, some as *ts'ang* (yin or passive) others *fu* (yang or positive).

To only stimulate identified points, following diagnosis, does not work for acupuncture as this does not correct imbalance by directly influencing yin or yang. In order for acupuncture treatment to be successful, it is also necessary to rebalance the body by

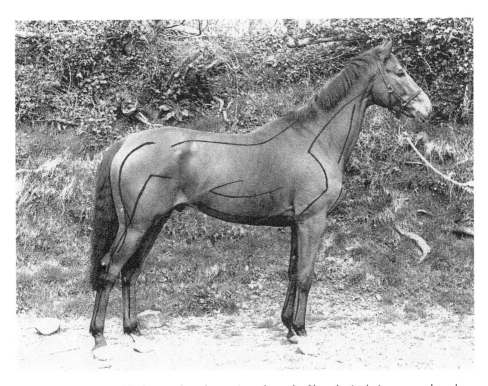

Fig. 10.2 Zone lines of the horse. These lines mirror the path of lymphatic drainage vessels and correspond to 'modern' meridians.

manipulating *ch'i* or energy. Because of the multiplicity of interactions between the body organs and energy, the stimulation of one point is inadequate and other harmonising, enhancing points will be selected.

Influencing a *point* is considered to affect energy flow, the energy will directly affect the organ associated with the point. Not only will the functions of that organ be activated, there will also be a knock-on effect, due to the interaction between all body components. The organ stimulated will influence and create activity within other organs which specifically react with the one first stimulated. Depending on the *ch'i* required (it may be yin or yang) and the type of organ, which in turn may be a *ts'ang* organ, those being relatively solid – heart, lung, liver, spleen and kidney – or a *fu* organ, these being hollow – small intestine, stomach, large intestine and bladder. The required effects can only be achieved by using appropriate point stimulation to initiate a complex chain reaction. The selection of points is complex. Choice must relate not only to the need to restore balance but also the interdependence of the whole, both within itself and within the environment, which necessitates consideration of the elements.

The five elements

Wood, fire, earth, metal and water are considered to be the primary materials from which the universe is composed. These five elements are not static, but are all continually passing through the processes of growth and metamorphosis. Their interactions create and destroy and this involves the transformation of both living and non-living materials. The lives of animals (and humans) also complete five changes which correspond to natural changes.

In the same way that starting to consider natural horsemanship requires a shift in the way you look at things, the philosophy of the five elements is difficult to explain in a literal, Western manner for there are no equivalent or comparable thought processes in the way we traditionally think in the West.

The concept of *creation* within the five elements is conceived thus:

wood burns;
fire creates ash;
earth results from ash, earth contains minerals;
metal is made from minerals;
water forms in a moist atmosphere, as a result of condensation on metal;
water feeds vegetation, thus completing the cycle as,
wood is recreated.

Destruction limits overproduction:

wood, the roots of the tree stretch into the earth;
earth is destroyed by roots absorbing nutrients;
water flow is limited by a dam, made of *earth*;
earth destroys *water*;
fire destroys *metal* by melting it;
metal shaped into tools destroys *wood*.

The fundamental rule is equilibrium. If any process dominates, be it creative or destructive, then balance is lost. Striving to maintain balance is of paramount importance. Even though acupuncture is conceived primarily as a means of maintaining health, diagnosis is required to ensure that the organs are functioning normally. Any deviation, however small, should be corrected before a yin/yang imbalance has resulted in malfunction or, as it is termed in the West, disease.

Diagnosis – Chinese principles

Even in a healthy animal, a decision regarding the points to be stimulated can only be arrived at after a step-by-step analysis of the animal's physical appearance as well as its demeanour. *Observation* is of paramount importance in Chinese veterinary medicine. As every horse adopts a different stance, be it at rest, standing, lying or while at work, the normal stance of a particular animal needs to be recognised before an accurate diagnosis is possible.

The four steps required for *diagnosis* are:

1 *Observation*:
   (a) lips: changes in lip colour are considered to indicate problems in the spleen and as the spleen and stomach are closely linked, lip changes also implicate the stomach.
   (b) urine: bladder problems
   (c) droppings: stomach and intestines
   (d) limbs: hoof problems (incorrect foot balance upsets limb balance)
   (e) skin: spots or pustules indicate blood and *ch'i* abnormalities
   (f) tongue: heart involvement
2 *Listening*:
   (a) breathing sounds: rasping, dry, stiff sounds all indicate lung disorders
   (b) grinding of teeth or crib biting are associated with kidney disorder
   (c) intestinal rumblings: Chinese veterinarians have classified each sound and related it to a specific area of the intestines

3 *Questioning*:

The owner is asked about appetite, respiration, droppings, urination, and the smell of breath, urine and droppings. The owner's observations are then related to the sex, age, size, breed and workload of the animal.

4 *Palpation*:

(a) general body palpation will indicate tender areas. These areas are noted, for each will correspond to a specific organ. Surface temperature and sensory responses are evaluated.

(The late Dominique Giniaux DVM, respected French veterinarian, had just begun to relate tender areas on the body surface to organs when he died.)

(b) pulse readings are taken from six sites on the front of the chest just lateral to the trachea (windpipe) – three on the right (the *three gates*) and three on the left (the *three portions*). The gates (*feng*, *ch'i* and *ming*) are associated with various organs, as are the *upper*, *middle* and *lower* portions.

Gate associations are:

- *Feng*: lungs and large intestine
- *Ch'i*: spleen and stomach
- *Ming*: *Ch'i* of the kidney and the triple burner (heater)

Portion associations are:

- *Upper*: heart and small intestine
- *Middle*: liver and gall bladder
- *Lower*: kidney and bladder

Each pulse is taken three times and each time the pressure is increased:

- *Fu*: lighter, superficial pressure
- *Chung*: medium pressure
- *Ch'en*: very deep pressure

Each of the readings is described by its quality:

- *Ping mo*: a normal, regular pulse, which in the horse at rest is 36–44 beats per minute
- *Fan mo*: a reverse pulse, abnormal in any one of several ways:
  - *Fu mo*: very 'light'
  - *Ch'en mo*: requires deep pressure to locate it
  - *Ch'ih mo*: slower than normal
  - *Shu mo*: rapid
  - *Hsien mo*: feels like a taut string
  - *Huang mo*: forceful
  - *Hua mo*: almost fibrillating, one beat 'rolls' into the next
  - *Sse mo*: intermittent, weak
  - *K'ou mo*: has a hollow feel
  - *Hsi mo*: feeble beat

To the trained practitioner, each of these reverse pulse findings indicates a state within the animal's systems. The location at which the pulse variation was noted will give some indication of the organ involved. Thus if the pulse taken at the *ming* gate is found to be *hsien mo*, then a kidney problem of obstruction involving both *ch'i* and circulation could be present. The correct points on the appropriate meridian need to be stimulated in order to adjust and balance the kidney and its associates before irreversible changes happen or disease manifests.

The pulses are considered so important that a further five *yie mo* (changed pulses) need to be appreciated. These pulses changes are *very* subtle and require great sensitivity of touch to appreciate the minute but important variations.

Yie mo or changed pulses are as follows:

- *picking pulse*: irregular rhythm with a missing beat after every third or fourth beat. Associated with a toxic condition.
- *leaking pulse*: feeble beats with an irregular rhythm. Associated with the heart.
- *entangled pulse*: feels very superficial and is intermittent. Associated with a toxic condition.
- *dashing pulse*: superficial feel, irregular and is felt as a rush then pause. Associated with gastro-intestinal problems.
- *puffing pulse* is reminiscent of the bubbles rising to the surface as water boils. Associated with failure within the five *tsang* organs.

Pulse appreciation is considered important for both diagnosis and prognosis.

The triple burner or triple heater

The triple burner is linked to the five *fu* organs. It has no single fixed anatomical location; nor is it entirely responsible for any specific organ. It is considered to influence functions, i.e. blood flow, lymphatic flow, *ch'i* movement, digestion, secretion and absorption. It is the transport and exchange stimulator. It is called *triple* as it is considered in three distinct sections: the upper, middle and lower burners each influence an area rather than an organ.

- *Upper burner*: facilitates body defence and lung function. The area is forward of the diaphragm and therefore embraces the front third of the horse. Included in this area are the lungs, heart, cranial thorax, neck and the head.
- *Middle burner*: facilitates digestion and nutrient delivery. The area lies behind the diaphragm and ends at the level of the umbilicus. The spleen, stomach and cranial abdominal contents are within this region.
- *Lower burner*: functions to maintain fluid drainage. The final third of the horse, from umbilicus to tail, contains the liver, large and small intestines, kidneys, bladder and organs of reproduction.

The appropriate sections of the triple burner require stimulation when diagnosis has identified malfunction in any of the functions it appears to influence.

Remember, the organs have their own stimulation points; the meridians are concerned purely with energy (*ch'i*) flow.

Modern western charts have extended the meridians relating to the horse and this has caused considerable controversy. In Oriental countries the points and meridian points described and used were compiled in 1972 at the Lanchau Veterinary Research Institute. The rapid increase in the use of acupuncture as an alternative therapy has led to confusion in application. There are many reasons for this. The romanisation of Chinese characters is not straightforward for there are several methods, each with a different system. Many romanisers failed to appreciate the subtle nuances of the various dialects. As many charts bear little or no relation to the original Chinese charts, it is small wonder that acupuncture has been a less successful therapy in the West. Undoubtedly, those practitioners who have remained faithful to traditional Chinese points achieve the best results.

Point stimulation

Traditionally, fine needles are inserted beneath the skin at selected points. The penetration depth varies depending on the locality of the point. Successful needle insertion gives rise to a definite response – as the needle sinks in the practitioner will feel a tightening around it. It feels 'steady' and will remain *in situ* without support. A loose needle which falls has missed the desired point. Once the needle is correctly sited, the acupuncturist will rotate it both clockwise and anticlockwise until an increased tissue resistance is felt as the needle becomes tightly grasped. Needles of various lengths and gauges are sold in sets.

In the UK, the Veterinary Act prohibits the insertion of needles into any animal by anyone other than a qualified veterinary surgeon. The low level laser can be used to stimulate points and finger pressure is equally effective. Learning to work with the fingers has the advantage of improving the tactile sensitivity of both the operator's fingertips and thumbs (an essential for successful massage) and as this sensitivity increases, an appreciation of minute temperature changes and variations in tissue tension can also be recognised, all of which are helpful when using palpation to aid diagnosis.

Laser acupuncture

Those who use low level lasers in a random fashion to 'treat' areas of the horse which they consider to be painful (for example, the back) are quite unwittingly stimulating acupuncture points.

Several, low level lasers currently available have multi-diode heads. The surface area of the applicator may be 2.5–4 cm (1–1^1/$_2$ inches) in diameter and to 'treat' a horse's back with such a laser and miss the acupuncture points would require considerable skill. Passing a laser with a multi-diode head down both sides of a horse's back from withers to dock could influence as many as 38 points. In view of the elaborate procedure undertaken by a veterinary acupuncturist *before* treating a horse, undertaken in order to ensure that the points selected will complement each other and achieve balance and harmony, then the activation of a mass of contradictory, rather than complementary, points is irresponsible. The lack of precision of the multi-diode head makes it inappropriate when an exact location is necessary for effective therapy. In this instance the more accurate, single diode laser should be employed.

Acupressure (traditional Chinese methods)

For *puncture* substitute *pressure*. Pressure techniques (*shiatsu*) are practised by the Japanese and the Chinese, who term the method of stimulation *tui nor*. The *acu* points are stimulated either by using small metal balls, a ball being placed over the point deemed to require stimulation, or by finger pressure. The balls are pushed down and inward with the palm of the hand, or left *in situ* on the surface and are held in place by adhesive tape. Small, spherical magnets mounted on bands are currently popular for pain relief in the human subject. It would be nearly impossible to attach effectively either a small metal ball or small magnet to a horse, particularly as the skin of a horse is considerably more mobile than that of the human. As explained in the description of point sites, points are located via skin resistance but if the skin moves, the underlying point will be lost.

The ball of the thumb is most useful for applying pressure to points, although some people prefer a fingertip or, for huge muscle masses, such as the muscle of the quarters, the point of the elbow can be used.

Effective acupressure needs exactly the same approach as acupuncture. First of all *diagnosis* should take place, leading to a consideration of:

- the selection of the appropriate points (5 to 15 are usually needed);
- the selection of the appropriate meridian;
- the consideration of yin to yang;
- the *ch'i* requirements.

Point location

It is impossible to practise acu therapies, be it puncture or pressure, without a chart depicting and numbering the points, the textbook relevant to the chart and an anatomy book. The relevant text to chart is essential, as each school of acu describes in a manner dependent on the original translation.

All points are described anatomically, for example, 'between the processes of T11 and T12', 'in the depression between the spinous processes of C1 and C2', 'in the fossa beside the junction of the scapular cartilage and the anterior angle of the scapula', hence the need for an anatomy book, particularly one which includes surface anatomy. The distance from anatomical landmarks is also carefully calculated: *tsun* is a measurement of length. The width of the 16th rib, at the point where an imaginary line from the *tuber coxae* (point of hip) crosses that rib, is considered in each individual to be one *tsun*. (Each *tsun* is divided into ten *fen*.) To calculate the *tsun*, a pair of dividers is placed accurately over the 16th rib at the appropriate site which will give a precise width which can be measured. The *tsun* calculated is appropriate for that individual only. In the point location chart the anatomical description will not only describe the anatomical landmarks but may also include two *tsun* from point x. In the needling/pressure charts two to three *fen deep* will denote a superficial point, while three to five *fen* denotes a deep point and needle or pressure must be applied accordingly.

Because of the variation in skin resistance over an acu point, finders have been developed. In effect, these are searching electrodes. The tip of the 'finder/detector' is sensitised to record the minute electrical variations within the skin's surface. When an area of lowered resistance is encountered the apparatus will emit a bleep or a light (usually red) illuminates. This all seems very simple, so why waste time with *tsun* and anatomical landmarks to locate acu points?

Due to the sensitivity of the apparatus, searching an area it will, unfortunately, pick up *any* skin change – a small patch of dried sweat, dirt in the coat or dampness. Changes will also manifest following local bruising or temporary compression, if the horse has been lying down, has had a tight roller or has been standing resting a leg.

The very mobile skin of the horse is a further complication, as tests on dead animals show the lowered resistance is only present in the skin, not in the underlying tissues, so a point 'found' by a point detector may not replicate the position in the deeper tissues. For accuracy, always double check using the anatomical landmarks and *tsun* measurements as described in the texts.

Point selection

Health maintenance rather than disease treatment is the purpose of Chinese medicine, and carefully selected points can and do influence body function, even when an animal is apparently in good condition. The selection of points will depend upon what you wish to achieve:

- Was the horse stiff after work?
- Is the urine thick and strong smelling?
- Is the horse restless?

All the steps described above in Diagnosis in the section on acupuncture (pages 88–90) need to be considered. Your decision must be carefully calculated, having determined the systems/organs/areas you wish to influence by a series of logical deductions after considering your horse as a whole. The points appropriate to the problem can then be selected by reference to the chosen chart and text. A London firm (Acumedic) stock a model horse with points marked and an accompanying text.

All basic texts describe around 114 points pertaining to the 'organs'. Each organ is governed by several points and each point will execute an effect fractionally different from other points which influence the same organ. No matter how small, that difference is critical when selecting a stimulation protocol. *Correct selection is the key to success and the only way to avoid failure.*

Meridian selection

Traditional Chinese medicine describes twelve meridians in the horse but only indicates one point for each meridian (see Fig. 10.3). This is unusual, as meridians are normally multi-point endowed. Westernisation of traditional Chinese medicine has extracted points from human meridian charts and allocated them to the horse, and in doing so the number of points has risen from 12 to 350!

Once the organ concerned has been selected, its governing meridian will need stimulation and its yin or yang requirements must be balanced by the release or containment of *ch'i* (remember, yin and yang cannot be influenced directly to regain their necessary equilibrium – this is achieved through working with *ch'i*).

Application of pressure

Suggested pressure requirements for different points are:

- superficial points = 5 lb of pressure or less
- medium-sited points = 10–15 lb of pressure
- deep-sited points = 15 lb of pressure

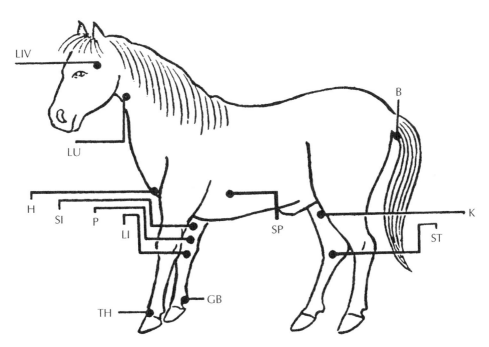

Fig. 10.3 In ancient Chinese charts, the meridians of the horse are illustrated as a single point rather than a line comprising many points.

The only way to understand your own strength is to experiment with a set of calibrated weighing scales. Using the finger or thumb, you intend to work with, push on the scales until you register the various weights suggested. You must then mentally note the sensation of thrust and transpose it to the pressure points.

While no type of point stimulation should cause the subject discomfort, occasionally resentment is apparent during stimulation or on the following day the horse may seem to be less comfortable than it was prior to therapy. Reappraisal is necessary in such situations. The techniques are supposed to be beneficial and while the benefits may not be immediately apparent adverse results indicate an incorrect diagnosis and or point selection.

Technique for acupressure

- The horse should be relaxed standing on a non-slip floor in stocks or in his own box.
- The operator should run their hands over the horse to accustom the animal to their touch and pressure. This is called *opening* (similar to effleurage, the opening and closing massage technique).
- The points must be identified accurately by feel or detector.
- Pressure is applied with thumb, finger or elbow placed not at an angle but perpendicular to the point.

Stimulation calls for the application of pressure at the appropriate poundage necessary for each individual point. The pressure should be applied using a small circular

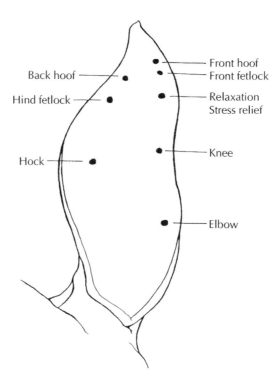

Fig. 10.4 Ear points after Giniaux and Westmayer.

movement. The time required for each condition will vary and should be indicated in your chosen text.

- Work the points from the head towards the tail and/or from the top towards the ground.
- After all the points have been stimulated on one side, move to the other, but *remember* some points are single as they are centrally situated.
- On completion of the second side, again run the hands over the horse as a final relaxation or *closing* (effleurage technique as for opening).
- The number of sessions required will depend on the results.
- Once a week is quite adequate as a 'top up' to maintain health.
- Over-stimulation wastes body resources.
- Remember the minute amounts needed in homoeopathic remedies.

Pulling the ears gently will also relieve stress. Ear points are marked on many early charts but are not documented in the book *Veterinary Acupuncture* (Klyde & Kung 1986) (see Fig. 10.4).

The late Dr Giniaux, considered several points beneficial and used several with success in stressed animals (see Fig. 10.5).

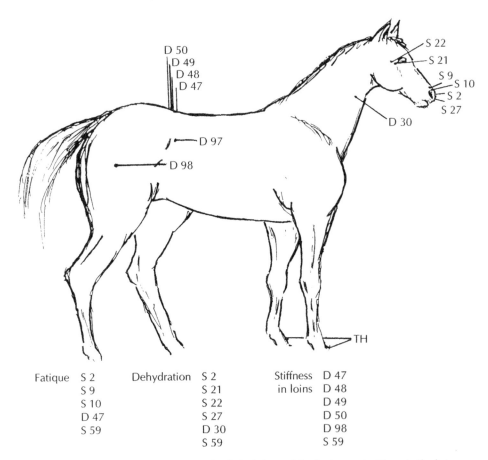

Fatigue	S 2	Dehydration	S 2	Stiffness	D 47
	S 9		S 21	in loins	D 48
	S 10		S 22		D 49
	D 47		S 27		D 50
	S 59		D 30		D 98
			S 59		S 59

Fig. 10.5 The location of points suggested to help fatigue, dehydration and stiffness in the loins, after Giniaux, taken from the *Chen Needle Chart*. S = a superficial point, D = a deep point. S59 located at tip of last tail vertebra. TH is considered the triple burner.

Points to stimulate for fatigue (Chinese), stress (Western) and the triple burner (see Fig. 10.5)

Point	Anatomical Location
S2 Bilateral	Three *fen* from the medial field of the nostrils on an imaginary line running from the lower border of one nostril to the other.
S9 Bilateral	Two *tsun* from the top of the nostril rim at its upper part.
S10 Bilateral	One *tsun* from the top of the nostril rim at its upper part.
D47 Single point	In the depression between the spine of the first sacral spine and last lumbar spine.
S59 Single point	The tip of the last tail vertebra (tip of dock).

Points to stimulate for sunstroke (Chinese), dehydration (Western) (see Fig. 10.5)

Point	Anatomical Location
S2 Bilateral	Three *fen* from the medial field of the nostrils on an imaginary line running from the lower border of one nostril to the other.
S21 Bilateral	On the transverse facial vein. One *tsun* behind and below the outer edge of the meeting of the eyelids.
S22 Bilateral	Five *fen* behind point 21.
S27 Bilateral	Three *fen* in, off an imaginary line between the lower border of the nostrils.
D30 Bilateral	On the jugular vein, junction of the upper and middle thirds.
S59 Single point	Tip of last tail vertebra.

Points to stimulate for muscle stiffness in the loins (see Fig. 10.5)

Point	Anatomical Location
D47 Bilateral	Two *tsun* in front of 48.
D48 Bilateral	Two *tsun* in front of 49.
D49 Bilateral	Two *tsun* in front of 50.
D50 Single point	In the depression between the spine of the first sacral spine and the last lumbar spine.
D97 Bilateral	On an imaginary line stretching from the dorsal midline to the tuber coxae point located on the lateral third of the line.
D98 Bilateral	Midway between the convexity of the trochanter of the femur and the patella.
S59 Single point	The tip of the last tail vertebra (tip of dock).

These charts described just three, basic prescriptions using the traditional approach. Although traditional methods have often been significantly altered to accommodate Western ideals, it does not mean they will not be effective. It may be that they are less effective than the original versions but the science has been adapted for twentieth-first century conditions. All science develops from basic concepts and all students need to appreciate the ground rules of any subject. Those who wish to pursue acupressure or acupuncture should, if they have grasped this section of text, have no difficulty in expanding their interests in either the traditional or the Western styles.

For those readers who wish to use acupuncture on their horses, appreciation of the complexity of the subject is perhaps best illustrated by the fact that the most recent veterinary text on the subject contains over 600 pages, of which over 350 are devoted to the horse. The method is not a 'short- or weekend-course' subject. Knowledge of the body functions, the ability to recognise behavioural changes, a precise anatomical appreciation and a precise diagnosis are all required. Treatment, preferably made by a qualified veterinary surgeon who specialises in acupuncture, is sensible, particularly when considering the fact that many of the cases seen today had no equal in the fifth century BC.

The early texts from which modern acupuncture stems, did not identify viral problems. Conditions such as gangrene, tetanus and convulsions have to all intents and purposes disappeared in the horse, however, laminitis, lung disorders and tendonitis still occur in the twenty-first century horse and many respond to appropriate acu therapy.

There are no short cuts in any of the complementary, as opposed to orthodox, therapies; all demand in-depth appreciation of the factors involved, including a knowledge of surface anatomy (see Fig. 11.4, page 108). Massage can and does complement acupressure, but it is also a subject on its own.

Further reading

All the titles listed below are available from Acumedic, 101–103 Camden High Street, London NW1 7NJ.

Essentials of Chinese Acupuncture, compiled by Beijing College of Traditional Chinese Medicine, Foreign Language Press, Beijing, 1980

Giniaux, D. *Soulagez Votre Cheval aux Doigts*, Pierre-Marcel Foure, 2 Rue du Sabot, Paris, 1986

Kaptchuk, T.J. *Chinese Medicine: The Web That Has No Weaver*, Rider & Co., London, 1983

Klide, A.M., & Kung, S.H. *Veterinary Acupuncture*, 3rd edn, University of Pennsylvania Press, USA, 2002

Schoen, A.M. (Ed.), *Veterinary Acupuncture Ancient Art to Modern Medicine*, 2nd edn, Mosby Inc., Missouri, USA, 2001

Westermayer, E. *The Treatment of Horses by Acupuncture*, Health Science Press, 1979

11 Massage

When compared to acu therapy, massage is a less complicated subject. It does associate with the former therapy, as can be seen by the requirement to open and close acu sessions by 'stroking'.

This section aims to educate readers in order to enable them to use appropriate Swedish massage techniques for their own horses, and to perform it both safely and effectively to enhance muscle function, a requirement of the ridden or driven animal living a domesticated existence.

There is some confusion surrounding the name, for although termed Swedish massage as though originating in Sweden, the principles and techniques are like those used in Chinese medicine, to enhance acu therapy. During the transposition to the West of the original Chinese methods of massage, French names were applied to the techniques, for it was the French missionaries who are claimed to have first imported massage. A Swede, Professor Hendrik Ling (1736–1839), then adopted the principles, and it is from these European interpretations that the techniques adopted became known as Swedish massage.

The principle underlying all massage techniques is the use of touch in order to stimulate nerve receptors sited both in the structure of the skin itself and beneath the skin, in the underlying tissues. The techniques described as Swedish massage form the basis of all other methods, no matter the name.

Good grooming undoubtedly has a massaging effect, many of the *syce* (grooms) in India, Malaysia and in the Middle East have a highly developed tactile sense, preferring to use their hands rather than brushes. Their charges revel in the hand contact, their coats shine and their muscles are supple.

Unlike a tracker in Africa, an Aboriginal in Australia, or a Dyak in the Malaysian jungle who touch the ground in order to calculate the time elapsed since an animal passed, or touch a tree, plant, fruit to evaluate its condition, people in the West rarely develop the full range of tactile senses available in their hands, for Western survival no longer depends on acute levels of dexterity and touch appreciation. As previously mentioned, natural horsemanship requires the search for, and improvement of, latent senses – learning to massage is an excellent educational exercise.

People who own and/or work with horses have often, without realising, marginally educated their tactile sensation, as they 'feel legs', test for dehydration by pinching skin, run their hands over the coat to evaluate its condition.

Massage might be likened to grooming with your hands, but it is much more subtle than that. Massage will enable you to 'join' with your horse, through touch, in a manner and depth almost unbelievable, honing the two-way man/horse interaction, until it almost replaces speech. Through massage, you also help prepare muscles for activity and enhance the body's own waste removal systems. Any assistance, such as massage, which does not require the body to expend energy is of the greatest value in the maintenance of health. Of course, activity increases circulatory movement, but activity requires energy, energy gives rise to waste, waste requires removal, energy needs to be replenished, replenishment leads to further activity. So, to describe the effects of massage as being only 'relaxation, pain reduction, increased lymph and venous return' is inadequate as these four factors have dramatic effects on the whole.

The wearing of a kennel coat, or overalls, even when working on one's own animal not only protects clothes but is also useful because horses are far more observant than they are given credit for. Once the horse begins to recognise the coat, it rapidly becomes associated with a pleasurable experience, leading to relaxation in anticipation. This should come as no surprise since the sight of the feed bucket or sound of the lorry all cause a predictable reponse in the horse.

The hands

Through massage, your hands become tools of communication. Correctly administered, massage should give as much satisfaction to the operator as it gives pleasure to the recipient, so ask a friend to act as the 'body', before experimenting on your horse, as they will be able to recount the sensations they receive from your hands.

You need to know or find out:

- Is the touch they experience comfortable?
- Can the 'patient' feel the whole hand?
- Is one hand working harder or deeper than the other?
- Is there too much pressure through the fingertips?
- Does the thumb pinch?
- Is there a nice rhythm as you perform the techniques?
- Does it feel as though an ant is running over the skin or do the sensations imparted lead to a feeling of confidence and security?
- Does the hand contact achieve a feeling of relaxation or create tension?

Have a massage from an experienced masseur yourself and enjoy the pleasurable sensations. Then have a massage from a novice – you will appreciate the difference. Experiencing good and bad techniques yourself will help you to massage well. When you change from human to horse, bear in mind that the muscle masses of the horse require greater hand strength to manipulate their bulk than do those of the average human subject.

Go slowly as a beginner – Rome was *not* built in a day. If you have difficulty in achieving rhythm, practise by using a body brush. Groom with the brush then replicate the grooming pattern by hand.

The secret of success in massage is to learn more and more about your hands; explore with them, mentally file all pertinent sensations and activities. In the novice this requires a conscious appreciation of exactly what you want your hands to do, the ways in which you need to use touch and feel, and what your hands tell you about the underlying tissues.

Running hands and fingertips over your 'friendly model' with your eyes closed will help you to learn the texture of superficial bone areas, limb contour and body angles. When you progress to the horse try to visualise the underlying structures, the lie of the muscles, build a 3-D picture of the whole in your mind.

Moulding the hands

Massage requires both hands to be moulded over the body surface, even if only one hand is working; the hands should be relaxed, with firm contact, exerting an *even* pressure. Various degrees of pressure during contact are required, just as with acupressure, the degree of pressure will depend on the form of massage selected, and/or the results required/anticipated. Pressure can be applied either by the hands, an elbow, fist, or finger/s. Spherical objects such as a tennis ball are used by some, but the information imparted through direct touch is lost.

Pressure

Variations in pressure will depend upon:

- the stroke or technique used;
- the effect required;
- the density of the underlying tissues;
- the presence of superficial bone points.

Rhythm

- Hand trembling, jerky movements, stops and starts and changes in rhythm will be resented and create tissue tension.
- Pressure should be increased and decreased evenly in a smooth flowing manner.

Speed

The rate of heart beat in a horse is around 36–45 bpm at rest. Work with this in mind when massaging. Rapid repetition, above the heart rate will stimulate rather than relax the subject.

Weight

Use your own body weight and movement rhythms as an aid. While your hands are the contact, exerting the expressive forces, the pressure is achieved by body rhythm *not by tense hands*.

Hands-on effects

As with all complementary therapies the effects achieved, whatever the technique, are not direct, but occur as a result of neural stimulation which triggers a series of chain reactions.

Massage reduces pain

Rubbing releases natural opiates. If you are kicked, you rub the area, the pain may not disappear but it does reduce; rubbing has resulted in the release of the body's own pain-reducing chemicals (opiates).

Massage achieves relaxation

A secondary effect of opiate release is relaxation and also a reduction in heart rate.

Massage warms the muscles

Manipulation of the tissues during massage increases the temperature within the targeted tissues. The body is programmed to remain at an ambient temperature, this requirement is controlled by the thermal regulating mechanism. The system is alerted to *any temperature change, anywhere within the body*, even a change as little as 1°C. Immediately a temperature change is registered, a chain of events occurs. The blood supply to the identified area is immediately organised in order to stabilise the temperature; in the case of a temperature rise, circulatory flow is increased in order to remove excess heat.

Massage affects arterial blood flow

Massage has *no direct effect* on arterial blood flow as arterial blood is under pressure and moves around the body due to the effects of the beating heart, the masseur *is not* directly pushing blood from A to B. It is the effect of the change in temperature within tissue that affects arterial flow, a rise increases arterial flow as the blood flow to the area is increased to restore the ambient temperature.

Massage enhances venous return

Venous blood relies upon the changes in pressure secondary to muscle activity for assistance in flow. Compression techniques mimic the pressure changes, within muscle masses, normally afforded by muscle activity, thus helping the movement of venous blood. As the circulatory system can be considered as a closed-circuit system, enhanced venous blood movement will have a knock-on effect through out the entire system.

Massage enhances lymph flow

As with venous blood, lymph makes use of pressure changes within the tissues to assist fluid movement.

Massage affects the nervous system

Massage techniques are applied over the surface of the body, the hands being in contact with the skin. The skin is attached to the underlying muscle masses by a tissue known as fascia. Fascia ensheaths all the systems of the body in one continuous interconnected, unbroken sheet. The main function of fascia is to support and stabilise the position of the various body systems. The tissue provides pathways for the suspension of circulatory and lymph vessels, in certain areas it affords anchorage for muscles.

Fascia is richly endowed with nerve endings (message receptors and transmitters) and it is this feature that is of importance to the massage therapists. The subcutaneous, fascial connection between the skin and all structures lying below provides, via the nerve receptors, a message relay system, enabling responses to any form of localised stimulation to be flashed throughout the entire body mass. Consider, for example, the effect of cold on the coat of the horse, living unclipped, in a natural situation. The thermal regulating system of the body is informed by messages from receptors specialising in temperature and sited in the skin and underlying tissues, when they are experiencing unacceptable cold. Messages are immediately flashed to each of the tiny muscles whose function is to raise individual hairs, the raised hairs of the coat trap air molecules and so create a layer of insulation.

In massage, many of the activated messages trigger reactions in areas distant to that being massaged. This is considered to be a chain response, the messages passing via the neural plexus of the *autonomic nervous system* previously discussed.

Acu therapy, trigger point therapy, connective tissue massage, skin rolling, the Bowen technique, shiatsu and Indian head massage *all use a variety of methods of touch application*. Some of these include body positioning; the changes in joint position, from that taken as the normal, involve/activate neural responses. Provided that they are correctly selected, these responses involve the entire neural control mechanism and can aid in the reduction of muscle spasm for example.

Muscle spasm reduces circulatory flow. A build-up of waste secondary to reduced circulatory flow leads to pain and pain leads to muscle spasm which leads to a build-up of waste – the vicious circle is established. All touch/pressure methods achieve their presumed aims as the result of stimulating neural responses, which in turn evoke chain reflex reactions.

If this is difficult to understand, then think about pain. Rubbing a painful area seems to help the pain, why? It is not directly because of the rubbing, but because the rubbing releases opiates made by the body, it was these and not the rubbing itself which reduced the pain.

Basic rules of massage

Swedish massage techniques are performed in the main in parallel to the venous blood flow. The two most readily available collecting areas for returning venous blood and lymphatic fluid are on the inner side of the elbow and in the groin, and it is preferable, if possible to direct strokes *towards* these areas.

If the coat lie allows, work in the direction of venous return.

- Start and finish with effleurage.
- Do not cause pain.
- If you increase tension rather than reduce it, change technique.
- If you use oils or liniments make certain that:
  (a) the horse is not allergic to them;
  (b) you do not 'blister' the area;
  (c) they do not contain prohibited substances (stimulants, sedatives).

Swedish massage techniques – effects and uses

For qualified masseurs of humans, several difficulties arise when presented with a horse. The horse is not lying down relaxed, and the masseur must work with the body mass in front of rather than below them, as when the subject is lying on a couch. Massaging the horse, as has been previously stated, is grooming with the hands. First, groom the neck with a brush then groom the neck with the hands.

Few people use their hands in an exactly similar manner, but this does not matter as long as the principle of tissue manipulation and the effects of the techniques are appreciated.

Effleurage (see Fig. 11.1)

In general, this technique involves both hands. They are moulded over the body contours, and contact is established throughout the entire palm surface of the hand/s, including that of the thumb and fingers. The hands may lie beside each other, one behind the other, or be wrapped around a limb, one above the other.

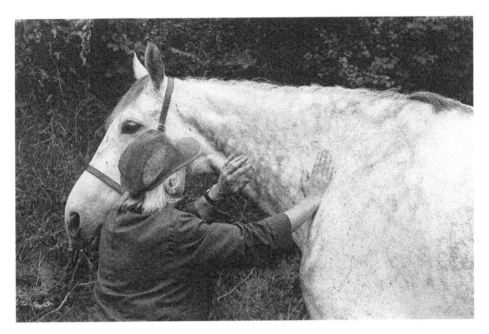

Fig. 11.1 Effleurage or stroking. The hand/hands mould to the body surface and the masseur performs a series of even strokes working towards the direction of venous return. The method is identical to opening and closing when performing acu techniques.

In massage manuals, the stroke is described as a long straight push, with the hands exerting the effective pressure as they are moved *away* from the body of the masseur. However, when working on a horse the strokes may need in some areas to be worked *towards* the masseur, rather than away, because of the growth directions of a horse's coat, and the fact that two available venous and lymphatic collecting sites lie in the elbow and groin areas.

- Pressure should be firm but not heavy until the animal begins to relax.
- Pressure can be increased as relaxation occurs.
- The final depth of compression should relate to tissue mass and location.
- The strokes should be performed in an even, rhythmic manner.
- A light contact must be maintained as the hands return to their starting position.
- After each completed stroke, the next is redirected until the whole area has been worked.
- Start and finish all massage sessions with effleurage, link varied techniques with effleurage.

Presumed effects

- Stimulates opiate release.
- Relaxation, leading to,
  - reduction of tension, leading to,
  - reduction of pain.
- Assistance to venous and lymphatic flow due to pressure changes achieved.
- Warms the tissues.
- Increased blood to tissues.

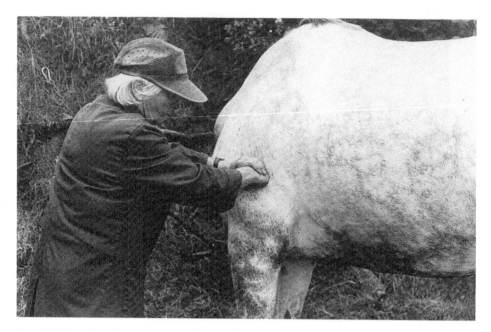

Fig. 11.2 Kneading, the movement is directed deep into the muscle mass.

Tissue movement increases tissue temperature and increased circulatory flow instigated by the body's thermal regulating mechanism.

Kneading or compression (see Fig. 11.2)

The purpose is to effect a compression followed by a reduction of compression, mimicking the effects of the alternating pressures generated within the muscle mass by contraction and relaxation of working muscle. The technique is used to affect tissue in large masses of muscle.

The working hand is positioned to form a loose fist. The back of the fist, the fingers and the knuckles are positioned over the treatment area. Movement is first directed downward, deep into the muscle mass. When both depth and required compression have been attained, the fist should roll in a slightly angled and upward manner to release compression. The movement sequence can be likened to that used when 'scooping out' deep frozen ice cream.

The technique demands some twisting (rotation) of the wrist and shoulder of the operative arm. As one hand tires the other takes over.

Presumed effects

- Compression of deep circulatory vessels within the targeted tissue targeted, leading to,
- enhancement of circulatory and lymphatic flow, leading to (if required),
- removal of waste and delivery of essential components.

Skin rolling

A double-handed, finger technique. A flap of skin on the neck is picked up between the fingers and thumbs. It is then *gently* moved using thumb pressure against slightly restraining fingers and as the hands move along the surface of the skin so one area of skin 'rolls' into another.

The skin can then be rolled back toward the masseur, with the fingers pushing and thumbs restraining. At the end of a movement, release the tissue and relocate the hands as required. The technique can be likened to the surge and collapse of a sea swell. The technique affects the subcutaneous fascia since this tissue is attached to the under-surface of the skin.

Presumed effects

- To stimulate superficial acupressure points (identical effects, various described techniques).
- To stimulate the autonomic nervous system (identical effects, various described techniques).
- Improvement of skin circulation.
- Stimulation of skin components.

Once again, we find interconnection between the 'natural therapies' of massage and acu methods.

Friction

Friction is a local technique when either the thumb or one finger, usually the index rein-forced by the second, is used to perform a deep penetrating movement. This may be *circular* or *transverse* across the line of the underlying tissue fibres.

- *Circular*: place the thumb or finger over the area and work in a series of small circular movements around or over the selected area.
- *Transverse*: this is performed most effectively with the tip of the index finger rein-forced by the second finger. The tip is placed over the fibres of the structure to be worked upon (the thumb can be used for a support). The tip of the finger is moved in a transverse manner back and forth across the damaged or scarred area. To be effect-ive deep pressure should be applied.

N.B.: The fingertip must *not* 'skin slip' – the underlying skin should move as one with the fingertip.

Presumed effects

- Creates a local hyperaemia (increase in local circulation).
- Irritates scar tissue and initiates resumption of improved repair.
- Irritates an organised haematoma and stimulates repair.

Finger massage

The fingers or a finger can be used effectively without involving the palm of the hand. Small muscles, for example rectus capitus and tissues sited in confined areas such as behind the knee, would be difficult to massage using the entire hand. Similarly, tendons, ligaments and the bulbs of the heels can be massaged with greater accuracy with the fingertips.

The hand techniques can be modified to fit this technique, but as the pressure applied will be to a small area, care must be taken to massage rather than to create friction.

Percussion, hacking or clapping

These are both two-handed techniques.

- *Hacking*: an alternating, double-handed technique. The edges of the little fingers of both hands are held just above the area targeted, then by twisting (rotating) first one and then the other forearm, the relaxed side of first one hand and little finger and then the second make contact with the body surface. In this technique, the masseur is aiming to deliver an alternating, short, sharp contact to the underlying tissue.
- *Clapping*: the hands are formed into a cup shape, both are placed side by side on the body surface. Using wrist movement, one hand is raised up, away from the skin surface, as it drops down so the other is raised. The hands continue to rise and fall in an easy rhythm until the entire targeted area has been worked.

Presumed effects

- Vibratory.
- Mild stimulation of underlying muscle.
- Stimulation of surface vessels.

The straw wisp, part of the grooming kit until straw became too short to plait, was used in a manner resembling clapping. The strapping pad has replaced the wisp and achieves an active process requiring energy as the muscles contract in reponse to impact.

In humans, the techniques are used to assist drainage in chest conditions. It has been suggested that application might assist a horse with a lung condition. *The inability of the horse to 'cough up' mucus from the lungs renders it extremely doubtful that these techniques have any place in assisting with problems concerned with equine lung conditions.*

General points for conditioning massage

Under normal conditions, most ridden animals walked at the start of any exercise. 'Walking the first mile out' prepared the horse for activity and walking the last mile home was the old way of enabling the horse to cleanse the by-products of waste from the muscles following activity. Even the naturally kept horse will, due to increased traffic conditions and reduction of good riding country in urban areas probably need to travel in a horse box or trailer in order to find safe hacking areas. While muscle activity is needed for balance when travelling, the warm-up walk should not be omitted. Massage is undoubtedly the best way of both preparing for exercise and restoring tired tissues after exercise (see Figs. 11.3, 11.4 and 11.5).

As with all techniques, the chosen approach needs to be appropriate both for the result required and *the state of the tissue.*

- When massaging locally, make certain the skin and underlying tissues move as one. 'Skin slipping' (skin sliding over underlying tissues) will create a local blister.
- If performing a general massage, work over the muscle groups which are always involved in normal activity; also select those groups required to undertake extra work, these groups will depend on the type of discipline the horse is to perform.
- Consider the direction of the muscle fibres and work *with* them, *not across* them, unless treating a condition necessitating cross-fibre work.
- If only using one hand, the free hand should be positioned on the body mass to act as a 'support contact'.

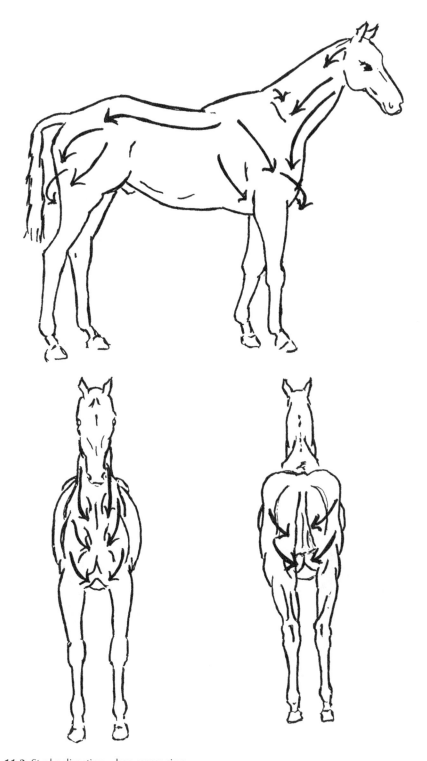

Fig. 11.3 Stroke direction when massaging.

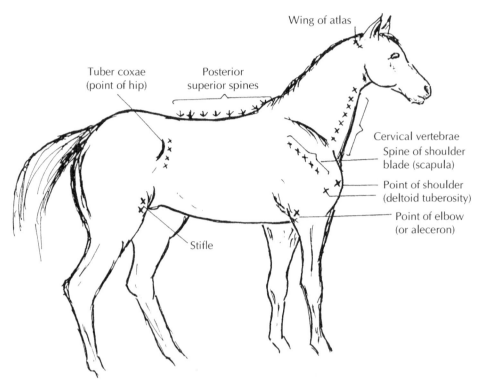

Fig. 11.4 Surface anatomy. Superficial bone helps to locate the definition of muscle masses. These bone landmarks are used to help identify points when using acu techniques.

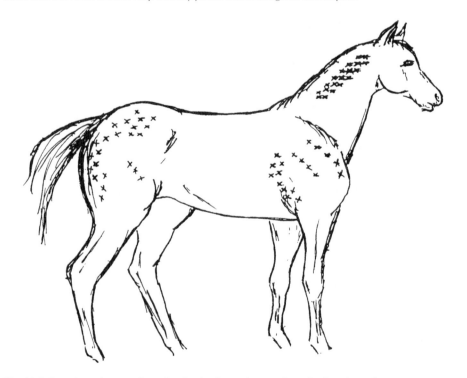

Fig. 11.5 Location of areas where the depth of muscle mass benefits from kneading.

Tension appreciation, finger sensation, touch

When at rest muscles maintain sufficient *tone* to retain the upright position, but they should feel 'soft', rather like potter's clay.

Muscles 'guard' damaged areas, whether the damage is to bone, joint, ligament, tendon or the muscle itself. The way in which 'tense' or 'guarding' muscles feel has to be learnt and a meaningful comparison sought. Increased tension will also occur if pain originates within an internal organ. Tension over the loins may be associated with the kidneys and most horse owners have seen the tightness of the abdominal muscles in a horse with colic.

What do you associate with the new sensation you have read through your fingers? As the fingertips become more sensitive, you will be able to feel the 'edges' of individual muscles, appreciate the presence of bone to which they attach, calculate temperature and changes in surface moisture. All this information contributes to the *reading* of your horse, every change in sensation is relevant. Even while massaging for health mainten-ance, you may discover the beginning of a problem, detecting changes in the feel of the skin and underlying muscles. Perhaps your hands discover an area of tension, the area also feels warm and/or damp compared to neighbouring areas, and yet you as the rider have not noticed a problem. Disruption within tissue increases activity, activity is a metabolic process which generates heat. Your fingers have told you something is wrong so search for the *cause*. There is rarely a problem without a cause and the problem cannot be solved unless the cause is addressed. *If you are concerned, talk to your vet.*

N.B.: Do not be fooled by areas of warmth which might have resulted from too tight a roller, the horse leaning against a wall, standing in the sun, or having been lying down, particularly if it was lying on a pile of droppings.

Starting

- Allow the horse to smell your hands. If you are using a gel or oil let the animal smell it.
- Run your hands over the neck, back and quarters to let the animal get used to the feel of your hands.
- Depending upon the type of massage required (general or specific) you should have decided upon the approach and techniques needed after an evaluation of the prob-lems being exhibited, i.e. stiff on the left rein, unable to achieve an outline, won't break from the stalls, etc.
- For other than a general toning massage, you must have a specific diagnosis.
- When the animal is used to your presence and the feel and smell of your hands, it is time to begin a planned session.

N.B.: Anyone can be wrong. If your plan does not seem to be effective, think again. It takes courage to admit to mistakes but it earns respect.

Finishing

After any type of massage always make a fuss of the horse and see it is comfortable. Finishing on a good note is as important as starting well.

General points when massaging

- It is preferable to work on a horse in its own box.
- Make certain there is nothing you might trip over if you have to move suddenly.
- Until the horse has learned to enjoy massage it should wear a head collar, and pos-sibly be loosely restrained.

- Occasionally, massage is painful and if the horse is tied and pulls back suddenly it may, in the future, associate restraint with pain.
- Remember that every horse will have a different level of tolerance.
- Every horse will react in a different manner to the various techniques.
- Some horses hate massage.
- In season, mares may be irritable.

Suggested routine

If possible, plan your learning massage sessions when the yard is quiet and there is little chance of being disturbed. Once your horse is accustomed to the pleasurable sessions it will usually arrange itself comfortably and wait for you to start no matter what is happening around you both.

Read your horse all the time, the signs of relaxation are obvious. The ears are very expressive, and as the horse relaxes, the head drops, the lower lip droops, the eyes become half shut, respiration slows. You may get a great deal of pleasure if the horse turns to rest its head on your shoulder or begins to gently chew your arm or shoulder.

As you massage, reposition your body slowly, trying to maintain a rhythm in tune with the strokes. Try not to tense your shoulders (you will tire quickly if you tense) and do not forget to breathe (people tend to hold their breath as they concentrate!). Effective warming of underlying muscle and relaxation normally occurs after ten to fifteen strokes.

Neck and shoulders

1 Position yourself by or just forward of the horse's shoulder, on whichever side of the horse you feel most comfortable.
2 Place your hands flat just behind the poll, fingers pointing upwards towards the top of the neck. Pull your hands slowly and firmly down from the top of the neck halfway towards the withers. Remove the hands and replace at your original starting point. Repeat several times until you feel the muscles relax (soften).
3 Direct the next pair of parallel strokes starting mid neck, downwards to the base of the neck, pulling the hands as before. Repeat until relaxation occurs.
4 Move slightly forward until you are positioned by the elbow. Direct the strokes from withers to the front of the chest by taking the hands downward. Repeat until relaxation occurs.
5 Place your hands on the side of the withers and direct the stroke down toward the elbows of the animal.

Two horses will often stand head to tail when in a family or companionable group. They communicate by gently chewing their companion in the wither area, sometimes just in front or just behind the wither. This area is recognised as a centre for communication – take advantage of this. You can work one side of the head and neck, then move to the other, or work the whole of one side of the body then move to the other.

The back

1 Position yourself just in front of the quarters on whichever side of the horse you feel most comfortable. (If the horse is very tall, stand on a milk crate.) Lean slightly

forward and place a hand on either side of the animal's withers close to the spine, with the hands positioned so that the fingers point toward the animal's head. Draw the hands slowly towards your body, exerting an even pressure. Repeat several times before going on to the next stage.

2 Moving the hands apart and repeating the strokes, gradually work further away from the centre of the back. The longissimus muscle stretches from withers to quarters and is approximately the width of one hand to two hands' span, depending on the size of the horse, from the middle of the back outward. Repeat as for stage 1 until the entire muscle in length and breadth has been massaged.

The quarters

1 Stay in the same position as when massaging the back, but turn to face the tail. Place a hand on either side of the top of the quarters with fingers pointing away from your body, and push the hands away towards the root of the tail.

2 The flanks and muscles at the top of each hind leg running up to the dock (hamstrings) are better massaged by first standing on the near side and then repositioning on the off side. To work directly behind any horse, however quiet, *must be done with great care!*

Near side quarter

1 Face the quarters and place your left hand on the loins for support contact. Place the right hand at the top of the quarters just below the jumpers bump (tuber sacrale) with the fingers pointing away from your body. Push the hand down and back towards the dock, then onwards and downwards to finish the stroke on the inner side of the second thigh (gaskin).

2 Place the hand below the point of the hip (tuber coxae), fingers pointing towards the stifle, and draw the hand downwards ending one stroke angling forwards towards the stifle. The following stroke should be angled towards the back of the second thigh.

3 Place the hand forward of the point of the hip (tuber coxae), fingers pointing upward, and *very gently* exerting a firm, but light, pressure draw the hand down towards the stifle.

N.B.: This type of work is often resented by the horse. If this is the case, abandon the stroke. Repeat the series on the off side quarter, working with the left hand, and using the right hand as the support contact.

Once you are adept, the total massage should take between 10–20 minutes.

Mechanical massage machines

Machine therapy is not a part of natural living, but an understanding of all features concerned with massage is useful.

Electrical apparatus, which are claimed to massage, do not supply massage in an exact replication of touch, rather the tissues are subjected to vibration. Many of the results are similar, but the operator does not have the benefit of reading 'through their hands' the effects of the therapy as happens when using the hands-on techniques.

The claims that the machines warm the tissues is correct, vibration/shaking results in tissue activity, activity results in a rise in temperature and the rise activates the thermal regulating mechanism increasing blood flow through the area of thermal increase. The frequency of the vibrations delivered by most mechanical massage machines is based on the work of Melzack and Wall (1996) who described, in their *Gate Theory of Pain*, the effects on neurons if tissue is subjected to cyclical vibrations, of a set frequency, over a set time. Melzack and Wall demonstrated a reduction in the ability of pain receptors to pass pain messages across a synapse in the main pathway leading to the brain. Result: no message, no pain sensation.

Reduction of, or cessation of, pain stimuli does lead to muscle relaxation with all the associated beneficial effects, including increased circulatory flow and loss of local muscle tension, but, and there is a but, it has to be established whether the tension was secondary to the pain stimuli *required to guard underlying injury?*

When considering the use of massage, remember that while hand massage can reduce pain, it does *not* remove essential guarding pain, unlike some other therapies.

Ice massage (useful for recent injury)

Tissue responds throughout the targeted area to cold application in the following ways:

- For approximately the first 15 minutes of application closing or constriction of local blood vessels occurs.
- There is decreased activity in local tissue reducing immediate oxygen requirement.
- Thermo-regulators (sensors) record and monitor the drop in temperature.
- As the ambient tissue temperature drops to an unacceptable low, the arterial circulation is alerted and a surge of 'warming' blood is dispatched.

N.B.: This safety mechanism will *not* operate if the temperature remains sub-zero for a long period as the sensors *cease to record*.

Ice techniques can be employed for large areas by placing ice cubes in a plastic bag (hand-held size), then massaging using a circular movement. The ice pack should be moved over the traumatised area for approximately five to ten minutes.

Local application to a small area

An individual ice cube can be rubbed over recent trauma in a circular manner. A supply of ice cubes with a 'stick' handle (iced lolly containers come in suitable sizes) kept in a deep freeze ready for trauma application is a useful tool.

Connective tissue massage

Each individual muscle is partitioned from its fellows by an outer sleeve of connective tissue or fascia. Look at a half leg of lamb at the next opportunity. You can plainly see fine white lines arranged around the masses of the red flesh of the muscles. The white lines are the muscle *sleeves* or *sheaths*. If you try to detach one mass and its sleeve or sheath from another you will discover that adjacent sheaths are interconnected, one to the other, hence the term *connective tissue*. Connective tissue massage is directed to these areas.

Connective tissue does not contain many elastic components. Should a muscle suddenly increase in bulk as a result of exercise, the connective tissue sheath may not immediately stretch to accommodate the volume increase. Stretch receptors will then record pain and muscle metabolism is hampered as the muscle attempts to work to increased demand and painful, ineffective contraction will result.

It is *sometimes* possible to relieve pain and stretch the affected connective tissue by directing a deep friction based massage along the lines of the connective tissue bands. *This is impossible without an extensive knowledge of the anatomical arrangement of the muscles, the organs, the skin, in fact every component that requires an adequate blood flow.*

Massage gloves

There are several massage gloves on the market. The operator's hand and fingers fit into a mitten, often made of flexible, synthetic, rubber-like material, the palm side of which may be ridged or covered in small raised 'bushes' like the soles of some golf shoes, or may have minute cone-like extensions.

The most useful are designed for the human rather than the horse. They are called 'bath mittens' and they enclose the hand providing a useful, light, easily moulded, slightly roughened surface giving a good grip and comfortable feel. They are particularly useful for gaining an animal's confidence, supposedly because the sensation may be similar to that experienced from the tongue or if the animal rubs against tree.

Technique

- Effleurage-type strokes are best suited to massage gloves.
- Incorporate glove massage with hand massage.

Underwater massage

The lower, or distal, part of the horse's leg often fill, as the circulatory return mechanism is poor. There are no muscles below knees and hocks to create the compression required by veins to function efficiently. The veins themselves, in the lower third of the legs, lack sufficient valves to ensure efficient venous return, particularly if the animal is static.

The frog, if able to function, aids fluid return to the body centre from the foot, fetlock area and distal cannon. Frog action is coupled to the movements of the sole of the foot. Both these activities are also dependent on adequate activity, foot balance, shape, health and trim. Neither action is fully efficient unless the horse has a correctly balanced foot.

The feral horse, unlike the stabled animal, is constantly on the move ensuring efficient venous return throughout the lower third of the limb, achieved by the constant pumping actions of the frog.

It is very difficult to massage the legs of a horse effectively and an old remedy handed down from the Romany Gypsies, who are reported to have rubbed (massaged) their horses, was to use streams to cool legs, horses were tied to a tree and left standing in the water.

The moving water creates variable compression, affecting the vessels which lie just below the surface of the skin and so aids the 'shunt' of venous blood. The cold also has a thermal, knock-on effect. As the limb temperature drops to below the ambient set by the body's thermal regulating centre, neural receptors signal the need for a temperature rise. The response is a sudden, arterial blood shunt within the deep limb vessels. This in turn increases local pressure, with a further knock-on effect within the veins associated with the particular arterial complex. The stream method also ensures frog action, the horse will become bored or uncomfortable after a while and start stamping.

Wellie boots (designed for front legs)

A pair of large, rubberised boots have a pipe in each toe leading to an air pump. The horse is persuaded to stand in the boots, water is introduced via a hose. Crushed ice can also be added for extra cooling. The water can be agitated by air delivered at the toe of the boot via the pipe connected to the motor. There is no danger of damaging the horse, as the boots are pliable. The boots merely fall over, spilling the water if the horse decides to move out of them.

Technique for underwater massage

1 Persuade the horse to place a leg in the boot.
2 Fill with water.
3 Let the horse stand and relax.
4 Add crushed ice if required.
5 Turn on the water agitator, and run it for ten to fifteen minutes.
6 Dry off leg.

N.B.: If the horse objects to standing in the water-filled container, hosing the legs first will nearly always achieve the desired result. Horses with wet legs are less reluctant to stand in water.

Massage routines

There can be no set massage routines or recipes, each horse's requirements will vary. There are many factors to take into account: the equine discipline, the rider's report describing the 'feel' experienced while riding, muscle contour, and details of any accidents sustained should all help to alert the masseur to areas which may require special attention.

The masseur should also be aware of the muscles subjected to unusual stress in each of equine activities and pay special attention to those muscles. Most often overlooked are the muscle groups concerned with adduction. In the fore limb, the muscles lie at the base of the chest and continue backwards between the fore legs to approximately a hand span behind the girth – these are known as the pectorals. In the hind limb, the muscles lie on the inner side of the upper part of the thigh stretching up into the groin. Vastus medialis, intermedius, sartorius and gracilis are all adductors. The last two are long, strap-like muscles, and both are partially inserted into the medial patella ligament, aiding stability within the stifle joint. The ligament is often highly sensitive to palpation and it is for this reason that it has been suggested that the ligament be considered within a general massage routine.

Once again, as discussed in all previous sections, success or failure rests upon an adequate assessment (*diagnosis*). In the case of massage, this assessment or diagnosis will be made by the masseur, enabling the approach most appropriate for each individual to be selected.

N.B.: Remember, tissue is alive and conditions change continuously. The suggestions in this section on massage, as in all other sections are based upon experience; they are *not* hard and fast rules.

Stretches incorporated in a massage routine must be selected carefully.

Muscles to massage pre- or post-exercise or at competition

In the past, most horses were groomed after being ridden, even if they had only been hacked out, many are now washed down. The suggestion that this may cause problems might be better appreciated by considering the following scenario. If you returned after a session in the gym or a run would you appreciate having several buckets of cold water poured over your body?

Strenuous exercise, whatever the reason, fatigues muscles and a massage given approximately two hours after exertion, when the horse has dried off, had a drink and eaten, will reduce the chances of stiffness the following day.

A massage session should start with five to eight minutes effleurage, and then be followed by techniques specific for the muscle groups involved in the specific discipline.

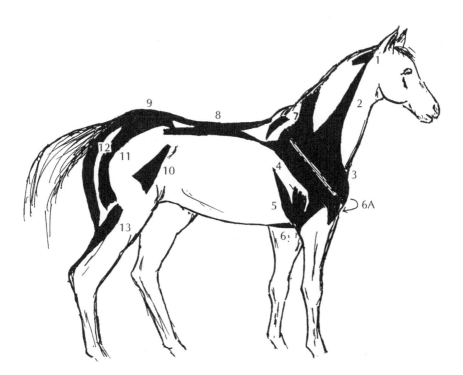

Fig. 11.6 Location of superficial muscles described in Table 11.1.

Techniques for deeper massage involve kneading, hand or finger usage suitable for the main superficial muscle groups are as follows in Table 11.1.

Muscle	Function	Technique
1 Rectus capitus	involved in stability of the head	gentle finger massage
2 Brachiocephalicus	involved in neck stability, if working singly turning the neck to the side	palm of hand cupped around muscle
3 Supraspinatus	involved in shoulder movement	localised finger massage
4 Infraspinatus	involved in shoulder movement	localised finger massage
5 Triceps	stabilises and works in all elbow movements	deep kneading
6 Pectorals	important stabilisers of the front legs during limb movement, work actively in lateral movements	knead gently
7 Trapezius	involved in the stabilisation of the shoulder blade/scapula	finger knead
8 Longissimus	suspension of the vertebral column from mid neck to pelvis. Back support when carrying rider weight	gentle kneading with fist
9 Gluteus medius	extension of the hip joint and so, hind leg	deep kneading, fist
10 Tensor fascia lata	stabilisation of hind leg, active in lateral work	finger massage
11 Biceps femoris	extension hind limb	knead/wring/finger massage
12 Semitendonosis	extension hind limb	knead/wring/finger massage
13 Gastrocnemius	extension hind limb	finger massage
14 Quadriceps	extension of the stifle joint	back of hand or fingers

N.B. 8 Longissimus: this muscle mass is often grossly diminished in horses in poor condition, if so, finger massage should be used.

Start and close with effleurage – time required, approximately 45 minutes. As a general rule, work on one side of the animal and then move to the other side. Regard the horse as a whole and keep the horse warm.

Massage, with veterinary agreement, is very useful for bruised areas following some types of accident. Its use is also beneficial following bruising of the back secondary to poor saddle fit.

The neck and back

Horses who fall when competing, get cast in the box, slip on a road, or lose, for any reason, their normal, four-limb balance will twist neck and/or back as they make frantic efforts to regain their feet. The exertions will stress the normal, balanced alignment of one or more areas of the back, the neck or both.

The trauma areas are easily located by palpation. Carefully palpate the entire length of neck from ears to withers and then the back from withers to croup. Incorporate the neck/back stretch routines as an aid to the location of the areas of trauma. Increased tension will be felt, with the muscle 'hardening' to touch.

Technique

- First use effleurage for pain relief and relaxation.
- Follow with local finger techniques to the areas assessed as being painful.
- Use general effleurage to close.
- Incorporate stretches *immediately* to prevent adhesions.
- Time allowed will depend upon the extent of the problem, but fifteen to twenty minutes is the minimum.

Bruising

Bruising is usually caused by the horse colliding with an obstacle while competing or as a result of being kicked.

A tiresome bruise may occur as the horse enters or leaves its box. This can be caused both by rushing and being too close to one or other side of the door frame. The point of the hip (tuber coxae) hits the doorframe and can be severely bruised by the contact. As there are a number of very important muscle attachments in this area, pain on all movements of the hind limb will result.

Technique

1 Ice massage the bruised area as speedily as is possible.
2 Follow with general effleurage to surrounding areas for fifteen to twenty minutes. Do this twice, if possible, on day 1.
3 After 24 hours, massage surrounding muscles using a general routine.
4 Follow by massaging the perimeter of the area of tension/bruising with the fingers, working towards the centre of the area.
5 Repeat the general massage to the surrounding muscle masses.
6 Treat daily until the bruise resolves.
7 Time required is approximately twenty to thirty minutes.
8 Follow with appropriate passive stretches.

Torn muscle

Tears within the architecture of a muscle occur if the fibres, often in a state of fatigue, are overstretched. The tears may occur near the origin of the muscle, in the main body (belly) of the muscle, or at the musculo-tendinous junction where muscle fibres begin to change their structural pattern to regroup as tendon. The amount of discomfort exhibited will depend upon the number of fibres involved and the secondary side effects.

When the muscle fibres tear, chemical activators are released into the tissue spaces adjacent to the tear. Their presence acts as a signal and the circulatory supply to the area is increased immediately. Unfortunately, the body responses tend to overreact and an excess of fluids arrives, only to accumulate in and around the damaged area. The increase in pressure causes pain and reduces the functional ability of local undamaged tissue.

Signs of a muscle tear

- Pain on palpation.
- Local heat.

- Swelling.
- Reduced activity of the muscle.
- A change in the way of going, often almost imperceptible.

Technique

1 Immediate ice application.
2 Ice massage around and over the area of damage 24–48 hours after injury.
3 Effleurage, working towards the elbow or groin.
4 As the swelling decreases (timing will depend upon the severity of the tear) begin to use the appropriate techniques, massaging daily until a normal pain-free state is achieved.
5 Use the appropriate passive stretches to avoid scarring after 48–56 hours.

Passive movements and stretches

Attempting to increase joint range stretches all other local structures, therefore, attempts to improve range are best done with the feet on the ground. However, this is not possible when stretching equine limbs and so the very greatest care should be taken when stretching activities are attempted. Unfortunately, many stretching exercises advised are described without the feet of the subject being in contact with the ground. It is essential, and the body expects it, to have ground contact experienced through the feet for perfect function, for the soles of the feet in all species are richly endowed with neural sensors. This is not only for balance, but also to initiate the body's own safety and conservation mechanisms. Consider these facts when choosing stretch techniques, if it is necessary to lose foot-to-ground contact, then ensure that the stretches performed are within the normal range for the joint or body area.

If a stretch is performed in a weight-bearing situation, the many safety mechanisms with which the body is endowed 'click in' and so avoid over-stretching. These mechanisms do not operate effectively in a non-weight-bearing situation. Non-weight-bearing stretching often leads to minor injury.

It is difficult to persuade a horse to stretch but it is perfectly possible to achieve by working it in long reins over poles, as the distances between the poles are increased so the animal must increase stride length, stretching all the working structures in a balanced manner in each of the four limb levers. It cannot be emphasised too often that great care must be taken when trying to stretch equine joints manually.

Some horses will stretch on their own, putting both fore limbs out in front of their body and bending down in a manner usually attributed to those trained in the circus, the liberty horses bowing to an audience.

Equine flexibility is just as important as rider flexibility and the ability of joint range is equally important in both species, but joint range is also associated with conformation. For example the horse with a very straight shoulder will never be capable of a very long stride.

Any form of stretching also needs to be performed when the subject is warm, no stretches need to be performed more than three to five times at any one session. The effect of stretching will not be instantaneous, it will take between three and five weeks to achieve increase in flexibility of the structures around the joints. To over-stretch in a hurry and try to achieve marked improvement in one session, is detrimental and causes micro-damage to the tissue architecture with consequent scarring and permanent loss of mobility.

Passive stretches are best given after massage, as they are designed to influence joint range as well as to increase muscle suppleness. They are *not* essential on the day of the competition. Their best use would seem to be during the period of fitness work given pre-season whatever the discipline.

Passive stretches should be performed *after* the tissues to be stretched have been warmed by massage. At the first assessment, *all* the stretches should be performed and the 'end feel' and range of each assessed. Those that require attention can be noted and incorporated in future massage sessions.

Despite extensive research into stretching in the human field, there are no definitive 'rules' only guidelines, the jury is still out with regard to the use of stretching. Currently, few human athletic training programmes are complete without the inclusion of a regime of stretching exercises, although in several recent scientific reviews 50% of the published papers considered stretching useful and 50% considered stretching afforded no obvious benefit.

Sports texts claim that stretching achieves suppleness of all the structures surrounding the joints and within the muscles moving the joints and that that stretching of joints and their supporting structures will ensure the full range of available movement is achieved and maintained. Logic suggests that joints are designed in a manner which allows for a pre-ordained range of movement. Trying to exceed this range by employing force is *not* the idea behind passive stretching. Muscles can be likened to finely tempered springs. If springs are kept well oiled they achieve maximum work with minimum effort. However, if they are allowed to get rusty and lose their recoil, the story is very different. It is possible that stretched muscles may respond like oiled springs.

The horse cannot be taught stretches and then expected to perform them by itself. Horses may stretch when they get up after lying down. They often tuck the nose toward the chest and stretch one or other hind leg backward. Some stretch both front legs forward after being girthed up, but regular stretching needs to be performed by the masseur. The owner or groom should be taught the correct procedure if appropriate.

General points

1 Tissues are less likely to tear or be damaged by overstretching if they are warm, so stretch *after massage*.
2 Study the anatomy of the joints before stretching.
3 Hold the limb in a manner comfortable for both you and the horse.
4 Position yourself so that you can move the limb without straining your back.
5 Never use sudden forceful thrusts.
6 Stretch slowly to the full extent of available range. At the first hint of resistance, stop, massage the resistant structures and try it again.
7 Stretch using a gentle traction. This will ensure that the elongation achieved will, in part, remain. Bouncy stretching (pull, release; pull, release) while increasing elasticity at the time, can cause a later loss of elasticity rather than an increase.
8 Repeat each movement five times.
9 Desist if the animal shows obvious resentment, or if the muscles appear to 'guard' by tensing.
10 At the end of *each* stretch allow the limb to reposition normally.

Head and neck

Full passive movement of a horse's neck by the operator is impossible to achieve because of the weight and resistance created by the tonic neck reflexes. Neck suppling is achieved with the aid of a carrot, polo mint or other gastronomic inducement.

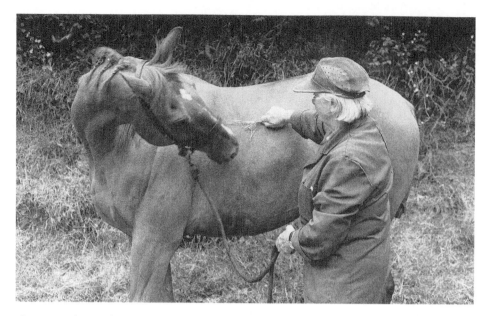

Fig. 11.7 Side stretch of neck. The horse is bending the neck evenly throughout, with very little head rotation.

Top neck stretch

Have the horse standing square wearing a head collar but not restrained, offer him the chosen bribe, slowly move it down his chest and then between his front legs. As his head follows your hand, so he will stretch the neck structures from poll to withers.

Side neck stretching (see Fig. 11.7)

Have the horse stand square, offer the bribe and slowly move it back towards his ribs. Repeat on the opposite side. A horse should be able to reach halfway down the rib cage with ease. Check to ensure that the neck bends evenly throughout. A badly tilted head or an inability to get muzzle to ribs needs investigation.

Check for muscle tension from poll to withers on both sides of the neck. Massage any hypersensitive, painful areas before any further attempts.

The shoulder

It is impossible to stretch the shoulder joint as an independent structure. The joint is part of a unit consisting of the shoulder blade (scapula) and the elbow joint – the site of articulation between the humerus and the uppermost bones of the fore limb (the fused radius and ulna).

The movements described anatomically are protraction (forward or extension) and retraction (bending or flexion). Both of these involve the elbow joint. Articulation between the hemispherical head of the humerus and the shallow acetabulum of the scapula comprises a ball-and-socket joint, so theoretically, rotation is possible. As the horse does not require such a complex movement, the muscle groups on the inner and outer aspects of the joint (the abductors and adductors) act mainly as stabilisers for the shoulder complex in the natural state. The lateral movements demanded in dressage require unusual activity in these two sets of muscles.

Protraction stretch I (knee at 90° angle)

1 Stand beside the horse, slightly in front of the shoulder, pick up the fore leg in the normal manner as if you were about to pick out the foot.
2 Transfer the hands and grasp the forearm allowing the knee joint to bend and hang loose.
3 Move the limb forward through its available range and then back to the normal position.
4 As the horse relaxes add increased traction at the end of each excursion of the limb.

Protraction stretch II (knee extended)

1 Stand well in front of the horse and slightly to one side.
2 Grasp the fore limb behind the fetlock joint and stretch the whole limb forwards and upwards to the end of range.
3 As the horse relaxes, gently increase the force applied at the end of the movement.

This stretch can be achieved by using a wide, woollen leg bandage (wrap). The unrolled bandage is placed so that its centre is behind the fetlock. The masseur holds the two ends of the bandage, pulling the limb forwards by the traction achieved as the bandage ends are pulled away from the horse. **N.B.:** This also stretches the knee in extension.

Retraction stretch I (knee flexed)

1 Stand beside the horse level with the shoulder. Pick up the fore limb in the normal manner as if you were about to pick out the foot.
2 Grasp the cannon bone and flex the knee.
3 Place one hand over the knee and push the limb complex backwards to the end of the available range.
4 As the horse relaxes increase the pressure when at the limit of backward movement.

Retraction stretch II (knee extended)

1 Stand well behind the horse's shoulder.
2 Grasp the forelimb around the fetlock joint.
3 Stretch the entire limb backwards and slightly upwards.
4 As the horse relaxes increase the pressure at the limit of movement both up and backwards.

Adduction stretch (knee extended)

1 Stand and position the limb as for protraction stretch II (above).
2 At full forward stretch, pull the limb outwards, away from the animal's body.
3 *Do not force* – stretch *carefully.*

Abduction stretch (knee extended)

1 Stand and position the limb as for protraction stretch II (above).
2 At full forward stretch pull the limb across the front of the body.
3 *Do not force* – stretch *carefully.*

The knee

The knee of the horse is a hinge joint. Its muscles and construction allow for flexion (bending) and extension (straightening) and small bones which comprise the joint glide within the joint during movement. Head-on slow motion films taken with the horse galloping demonstrate the entire limb rotating in mid-air flight as the fore limb stretches forward with the foot feeling for the ground.

The knee joint cannot be manually stretched to full extension. Protraction stretch II achieves extension but is approximately 15° off full extension.

Knee flexion I

1 Stand beside the horse and grasp the cannon bone.
2 Bend the knee until the back of the fetlock touches the underside of the forearm.
3 The forearm must be parallel to the ground.
4 Move the cannon bone inwards until the back of the fetlock is no longer in contact.
5 Push the cannon gently upwards.
6 Repeat but pull the cannon outwards.

Ten to fifteen degrees of extra movement will be achieved.

N.B.: Some horses have restriction of these movements following knee surgery, or if arthritic changes have occurred. In these cases stretch *very carefully.*

Knee stretch II

1 Proceed as for knee flexion I (above).
2 Stop flexion approximately 15° before the back of the fetlock touches the underside of the forearm.
3 Push the cannon towards the centre of the body, then pull outwards away from the centre of the body.
4 *Never force knee movements.*

Fetlocks

The extension excursion achieved within the fetlock joints of both the front and hind limbs, when either limit is fully protracted and the entire body weight of the animal is supported on the limb, cannot be achieved manually.

Fetlock stretch

1 Stand and grasp the limb exactly as when picking out the foot.
2 Hold the foot in one hand and the cannon above the joint in the other.
3 Move the foot up and down with overpressure at the end of each movement.

The hip joint

The hip is a powerful ball and socket joint (see Fig. 14.3, page 146), like the shoulder joint, but the hip joint exhibits a construction design of considerably greater strength, with a deep, bowl-type socket (acetabulum) containing the massive, half-spherical femoral head. The femoral head is attached by an internal as well as by external ligaments. The movements at the joint are primarily flexion and extension. Body mass, muscle and ligament placement limit range to ensure safety and strength.

The hip, stifle and hock joints must be considered as a single unit. Stretches of the individual joints are not possible. The complexity of the unit and its function during motion demand levers as well as the associated muscle power and excursion. Safety and limitation of movement are partially achieved through ligament length. While the hip is an independent joint within the complex, hock and stifle movement are coupled together. Flexion or extension in either one of the two immediately causes the same movement to occur in its partner. This feature is ensured by virtue of tendinous bands within local structures, in particular, peroneus tertius. The movements within the complex are also dependent upon the stability of the stifle joint. Problems such as 'stifle locking', or orthopaedic disease such as cystic conditions, transmit extra strain upon the hock joint, which is the hardest working joint in the horse.

Hind limb stretch I

1 Stand level with the midline of the horse, facing towards the tail.
2 Grasp the limb at mid cannon and pull the limb forwards and up.
3 When the horse settles, increase the traction force.

Hind limb stretch II

Do not attempt this stretch on any horse known to kick.

1 Stand behind the horse, slightly to one side, facing the quarters.
2 Grasp the cannon bone and pull the limb complex backwards.
3 If the horse settles, increase traction at the end of movement range.

The range of movement in the joints of the hind limb is less than those of the front limb. Neither hip, stifle or hock can extend to a 90° angle, and flexion is limited by construction and body mass.

The back

The horse's back needs to be stable rather than highly mobile. It is interesting to note that during activity the two sections which are subjected to the greatest movement stress are the junction of neck to chest and the junction of vertebral column to pelvis. This is completely different to man in whom stability at the base of neck and junction of loins to pelvis is essential. It is always worth reflecting on the fact that there are notable variations between the species and that what works for man may well be inappropriate for the horse.

The horse's back is generally considered by horsemen to stretch only from withers to loins, the area over which the saddle sits. Remarkably little attention is paid either to the anatomical features or to the biomechanics, but the back should be always be considered in conjunction with the neck and loins rather than in isolation. The isolated approach, may, in part, be due to the widely differing opinions of the experts and there is just as much confusion regarding the human back!

There are known movements in the area of back which carries the saddle. They are described in anatomical terms as the following:

- flexion: rounding the back, creating a dorsal convexity. To the rider this is known as 'lifting'.
- extension: hollowing the back, creating a ventral convexity. To the rider this is known as 'going hollow'.
- side bending, side flexion.

Certain movements demand axial rotations. The construction of the horse allows for this, for if rotation was blocked, then the components would break (fracture) under the strain.

Although movement is present, the horse *does not* perform any back movements as a regular voluntary action. He will bend his neck sideways to bite his sides if troubled by an irritation, and if the irritation is on his flank he stretches his hind limb forward towards his bent neck. The horse may also attempt to influence back pain by rolling or kicking back, and when mounted by bucking, but does not stand in a field or box deliberately exercising its back as a daily activity by rounding, hollowing or bending sideways. However, if the correct reflex areas are stimulated then the movements occur as a *reflex response*.

Consider the horse's back as a sprung girder with minor collapse and recoil available to absorb the concussion generated during movement as the limbs meet the ground. Anatomically, the back begins not at the withers, but between the shoulder blades at the site of the first thoracic vertebrae. A main part of the suspension system lies between the front legs where the forward ribs attach to the breastbone (sternum). Problems within this complex will affect the entire back, for the greatest amount of dorso-ventral movement occurs in two areas: at the first thoracic vertebral complex just described and at the junction of the loins to quarters, the lumbo-sacral junction.

Recent work in Japan (private comm.) using implanted electrodes to monitor the muscle activity of the back during walk, trot, canter and gallop over ground with and without a rider, demonstrates differences both in movement range and in the muscle firing patterns. The added rider weight causes some muscle groups to adopt a partially static, rather than a fully active role. The work, still in its early stages, suggests that for the back to work when ridden, in a manner which mimics that of the riderless horse, requires great attention to saddle fit. This is not a new concept. Smith (1891) wrote a treatise on saddle fit and designed the cavalry saddle which is still in use over 100 years later. Rider weight needs to be distributed over as large an area as is practical via flat panels which mould to the contours of the equine back. The gutter between the panels bridging the center of the back should be wide, allowing for recoil and thus shock absorption within the bone complex of the spine.

Back stretches cannot be performed passively by the masseur, but movements of the back can be achieved by stimulating reflex points. The horse must be relaxed, preferably following a massage session, to induce the required responses. It is not only the limb joints which require flexibility. It is essential in the neck joints and probably the tail; little is known about the manner in which the tail aids balance, but it is certainly not there just to flick off flies. For example, the horse raises its tail to initiate a closed-chain reflex which braces the hind legs just before it takes off to jump, it also tucks its tail in to increase tension in the musculature of the croup and loins before bucking.

A horse which clamps its tail while working will tend to have a stiff hind leg action. Clamping is therefore an indication of discomfort in the croup/loin area. The animal clamps to ensure that muscle activity, which might cause pain through movement, is restricted to a minimum.

Gentle tail circling relaxes the hind quarters and back, most horses seem to enjoy this method and Linda Tellington Jones incorporates the technique in her routines with great success.

Rounding

1 Stand with one hand on the withers and place the other hand on the centre line just behind the girth and just forward of the umbilicus.
2 Press firmly upward. The horse will raise his back and lower the head.

Hollowing

1 Stand by the side of the horse.
2 Run the hands along the back, one on either side of the centre about one hand's span from the centre.

3 Position the hands forward of the loins, approximately where the rider's seat bones would meet the saddle if it were in place.
4 Press firmly down.
5 The horse will hollow the back and raise the head.

Side flexion

1 Run the tips of the fingers along one side of the back from withers to loins a half-hand span from the centre of the back.
2 Press firmly as the fingers move back towards the quarters.
3 The horse will bend away from the pressure.
4 Repeat on the opposite side of the back.

Desist if the horse shows any resentment to pressure or if the muscle goes into spasm to 'guard' an area. This reaction indicates there is a problem which needs to be addressed.

It is interesting to note that the head raise/back hollowing reflex can be activated by the pressure caused by a rider sitting too deep. The horse is forced to dip the back and raise the head as the result of a reflex over which is has no control – its brain makes this occur as an automatic response. When this happens, the position of back and neck is incorrect and outline is lost.

All too often, instead of addressing saddle fit and rider weight distribution, a restraint designed to lower the head by pressure on the sensitive bars of the mouth and/or on the sensitive poll is used to force the head down. Small wonder the animal becomes confused: its brain is giving one command, and the pain it feels is giving another conflicting signal, with tension as the immediate result. When this occurs, the animal cannot work in a relaxed supple manner.

To achieve flexibility by passive stretching requires time and patience. Conformation must be considered, along with muscle build. Do not expect exactly similar responses from each animal – after all, not all humans can touch their toes with ease!

Do not 'overdo' the routine. The concept that 'the more the exercises are done the better' is false. Enough is enough, too much is bad. It is better to do too little than too much. It will take approximately three weeks before any improvement in tight structures is observed. Once this is achieved a weekly maintenance stretch will be sufficient to retain flexibility.

To recap, muscles are similar to groups of beautifully tempered, balanced springs. Your horse depends upon healthy muscles for effective movements and healthy muscles require a strong bone structure both to act as a leverage system and as an anchor for muscle attachment. Other essentials are systems for command, delivery of food, removal of waste, repair facilities, and temperature control.

Summary

You can aid your horse by ensuring that it has access to a dietary intake as palatable, natural and well balanced as is possible to ensure both general and muscle health. Through the use of massage and passive stretching you can help muscles, which in a natural state are continually active, to remain pliable and therefore efficient in the unnatural lifestyle most horses have been forced to adopt through domestication. Evolutionary changes do not occur rapidly – horses still need space to run free if they so wish.

Further reading

Chaitow, L., DeLany, J. & Peters, D. *Modern Neuromuscular Techniques*, Churchill Livingstone, 1997

Field, T. *Massage Therapy Research*, Churchill Livingstone, 2006 (www.elsevierhealth.com)

Holey, E.A. & Cook, E.M. *Therapeutic Massage*, 3rd edn, W.B. Saunders & Co, London, 1998

McBride, S.D., Hemmings, A. & Robinson, K. 'A Preliminary Study on the Effects of Massage to Reduce Stress in the Horse', *Journal of Equine Veterinary Science*, Vol. 24 (2), pp. 76–81, 2004

Meager, J. *Beating Muscle Injuries for Horses* (self published), 1985

Melzack, R. & Wall, P.D. *The Challenge of Pain*, Penguin, London, 1996

Meyer, T. *Sportmassage*, Copress Verlag, Munchen, 2005

Smith, F. *A Manual of Saddles and Sore Backs*, Army Veterinary School, Aldershot, 1891

Part III

Training/Building The Horse

Books on training the horse often describe activities thus, 'do this exercise and your horse will become supple'. So, why does your horse become supple, what are the reasons?

To illustrate with a human example, everyone is told how to lift a weight to avoid back injury, 'bend the knees and hips, keep the back straight, lift with the weight close to the body'. Why? Does the text explain how to put the weight down? The author has not as yet been able to find in any lifting guide the reasons for lifting in a certain manner to save the back, nor, with the reader left holding the weight after lifting, is there any described method of putting it down to save the back. Might there be, for example, specific exercises that should be used to target and so strengthen the muscles used when lifting, if so what are they?

If your horse finds a movement difficult, what is the reason? If there are no veterinary/lameness problems, could it be lack of appropriate muscle building? The answer to this is probably. This section of the book, 'Training/Building the Horse', aims to explain sequential muscle building which will enable the reader to understand the reasons for it and why it is important. The section, Suggested Exercises, describes the muscles/muscle groups targeted by the exercises/activities. This is to allow the discerning reader to analyse the muscles involved in the movement which their horse is finding difficult and then, by choosing the appropriate activity, target the identified areas of weakness.

The secondary effects of training specific muscle groups and the results that the rider may expect in overall performance are also suggested.

Muscle is slow to adapt to cope with increased demand, the description of the body systems earlier in this text has indicated some of the complexities. Before considering total body training it is necessary to consider some of the terminology associated with muscle activity and the implications of the different activities. Only by doing so is it possible to plan appropriate programmes for improved performance, and to make intelligent use of the many books discussing exercise. Although these books have mostly been written in regard to human activities, this is an area where for a considerable time it has been appreciated that different activities each require a specialist protocol.

12 Terminology Associated With Muscle Activity

Terminology is not as specific as might be hoped. The terms condition, conditioned and fitness tend to be used indiscriminately, both when discussing the state of the horse in question and level of training achieved. 'In good condition' suggests good general health. Muscle, if trained and ready for specific tasks, even just general riding, is described as conditioned. Fitness encompasses both the cardiovascular state and the level of exposure to the task required. The aim of training should be to produce a well-conditioned, fit horse.

The terminology associated with muscle and activity deserves consideration:

- *Condition*: muscle condition is the state of muscle. It can be soft (not ready for strenuous activity); toned; conditioned.
- *Conditioned*: appropriate demands, by nature of graded exercise, have activated and prepared all the systems involved with muscle function.
  These include:
  - Improved neural response.
  - Improved employment of motor units within each individual muscle.
  - Adequate circulation involving proliferation of the capillary bed.
  - Adequate fuel loading.
- *Tone*: exercise improves muscle condition, the 'tone' (state) improves.
- *Capability*: activity (exercise) both conditions, and improves muscle capability. The muscles become capable of performing the required task without undue or early fatigue onset.
- *Loading*: systematically increasing the levels, or the demands of work, in order to further improve muscle capability. Loading includes increasing the resistance encountered by working muscles.

Muscle function

As previously stated, muscles use the bones of the appendicular skeleton as levers, but no lever can work without a fulcrum. Due to the complexity of the equine skeleton, each muscle is required to fulfil a variety of specific, named roles. No muscle ever works as a single entity or uses its full contraction capability at any one time, the number of contractile or motor units activated should be sufficient to achieve and complete the demands of the required task. Over a period of time, as the activated units tire, others imperceptibly take on the task, allowing the by now fatigued fibres time to cleanse and reload with fuel.

Understanding the effects and results of varied muscle activity will enable the trainer of the domesticated animal to choose appropriate activities to build muscle.

Group activity of muscles

- *Prime mover (agonist)*: the muscle which initiates the first activity leading to a chain of events.
- *Antagonist*: works in opposition to the prime mover ensuring a smooth movement. The muscle lengthens or pays out when the prime mover shortens, or the muscle shortens if the prime mover lengthens.
- *Secondary agonist*: a muscle group which may need to be recruited to assist the prime mover if the task demanded is too great for one group of muscles.
- *Secondary antagonist*: the muscle works in opposition to the secondary agonist ensuring smooth movement.
- *Stabiliser or fixator*: a muscle, or group of muscles, acting to form a stable, temporarily immobile area affording the prime mover an anchorage to effect the required movement.

Muscle actions are described as follows as there are different types of contraction:

- *Concentric muscle contraction*: the muscle reduces its resting length, or shortens to achieve movement. Efficient and economic.
- *Eccentric muscle contraction*: the muscle becomes actively engaged as the prime mover, but does not shorten, the tissue lengthens during activity while loaded, to effect the movement required. Example, the fore limb stretching forward on a downhill slope. This type of muscle work is very demanding, particularly if muscle is unprepared for tasks necessitating eccentric work.
- *Synergic muscle contraction*: muscles are working in harmony with all interacting groups during movement ensuring economy of effort by eliminating unnecessary, or excess activity.
- *Static muscle contraction*: muscles have to achieve a working tension but are unable, by virtue of the demanded task, to contract or relax. They fatigue rapidly.

  Dressage demands a great deal of static work as the animal 'holds an outline'. It is the most exhausting of all types of work for the tension created reduces the ability of the muscle to cleanse and also affects the delivery of much-needed fuel.
- *Active muscle contraction*: a muscle working actively contracts, increasing tension within the mass, and then relaxes, reducing tension within the mass. These constant changes of tension within the muscle influence circulatory flow, particularly venous return, allowing waste removal.

  Arterial flow increase, required for delivery, occurs in response to signals initiated by the demands of working muscle.

  Active muscle work therefore increases circulatory flow and results in calculated responses necessitating increased activity in the cardiopulmonary system involving the heart and lungs.

While it would seem reasonable to assume active work is the prime cause of fatigue, it is in fact less fatiguing than static work. It is for this reason that if a horse is asked to hold an outline during flat-work schooling sessions, the head and neck should be frequently released and the horse allowed to stretch.

The increased tension within a muscle may be:

- *Isometric*: the working muscle or group functions by increasing tension but not shortening.
- *Isotonic*: the working muscle or group anticipates the function and contracts slightly to achieve a state of readiness.

Range of motion

The movement of one bone against another occurs at their place of connection or joint. Movement of the body occurs, as previously stated, when muscles recruit the bones of the appendicular skeleton and convert them to levers. The range of lever angulations possible will depend upon the anatomical shape of joints as well as on the flexibility of the soft tissues passing over them. The combination of these two factors controls the amount of movement which can occur between the bones forming a joint. The full movement possible at any joint is termed the range of movement.

As the joint or joints move through their range of motion, all the structures which service the area are affected – the joint surfaces, joint capsules, ligaments, blood vessels, nerves, lymphatic, and of course the muscles themselves.

Movement is described using terminology applicable to joints:

- flexion – bending;
- extension – straightening;
- adduction – moving towards to the body;
- abduction – moving away from the body;
- rotation – turning.

Muscle range is related to the functional activity of the joint or joints over which an individual muscle passes. Muscle range is taken to be the distance from complete elongation of the muscle to maximal shortening of the muscle.

Imagine a geometric protractor; the lever to be moved lies along the 180° base line and the line is broken at the 90° angle. A simple example is to consider the human elbow. When the arm is straight, the biceps or 'bending' muscle is fully elongated. If measured using a protractor, the full stretch angle at the elbow joint is 180°. As the muscle shortens, the elbow bends or flexes passing through a 90° angle until, due to both the construction of the elbow joint and the fact that the muscle bulge of both forearm and upper arm meet, the bending at the joint is fifteen to twenty degrees off the complete range described on a protractor.

Arc of movement

Different actions call for muscles to work within three ranges and movement is broken down descriptively, with the 'full range or arc' being subdivided into three:

- inner range;
- middle range;
- outer range.

Each range places a different load on the working muscle. Once this fact is appreciated it becomes possible, when planning training, to vary the work requirement of muscle by changing the pattern of limb excursion. Change of limb excursion will also vary the range of movement at joints.

- *inner range*: the muscle works through a decreasing 45° angle, this ensures stability but with little movement range in the supported joints. The postural muscles employ this range.
- *middle range*: described as the arc of movement from approximately 145° to 45°. Work in this range is an excellent way to improve muscle capability.

- *outer range*: the arc of movement is described as being from 180° to 145°. This range is economic, with the muscles assisted by elastic recoil from the ligaments sited around the moving joints. Stretched during joint movement, they load with kinematic energy, the release ensures the ligament reforms to the pre-stretch configuration. Outer range is the preferred range adopted, for economy, by the natural horse.

If allowed, a horse will 'run', using outer range, rather than work, using middle range, particularly if being worked on a lunge by an inexperienced handler.

Muscle fibre types

Three fibre types have been identified within the composition of skeletal muscle in the horse. They are classified by differences in the speed of contraction and by their varying need for oxygen. All breeds exhibit all three fibre types but in differing proportions (Snow & Vogel 1987).

There appears to be a genetically inherited predominance of fibre type. For example, the flat horse has been selectively bred for speed over a short distance requiring a pre-dominance of fast twitch muscle. However, even with careful selection, one individual in a family may be endowed with a higher proportion of speed ability than a brother or sister in whom the genetic mix, despite selection, is dissimilar.

Speed is multifactorial and to change a horse to another discipline, such as dressage, using an animal bred and trained to go very fast over a short distance, takes years not months. The different discipline requires the use of a totally different pattern of muscle activity, with recruitment of the available, predominately dormant, slow twitch fibres.

Slow twitch fibres

These types of muscles have a complex but very efficient energy usage which requires oxygen. As the name implies, not only do the muscle fibres contract fractionally slower than fast twitch type muscle but slow twitch muscles fibres are also capable of prolonged periods of activity. They can be considered as endurance fibres like those required by the long distance runner. The endurance horse requires a predominance of this fibre type and despite the fact that all muscles are a mix, training methods can be adjusted to involve the recruitment of a greater percentage of the fibre type best suited to the task.

Slow twitch fibres (ST), (slow oxidative (SO))

- These fibres contract slowly and relax slowly.
- They are dependent on oxygen for efficient function.
- They are able to store fats as a source of energy.
- They store relatively little glycogen.
- They have a reddish appearance as a result of their rich blood supply.
- They are bulky.
- They are stamina fibres.

The tissue of these fibres responds to long periods of slow, steady work, gradually involving an increase in distance.

Fast twitch fibres

Fast twitch fibres enjoy a slightly different chemical fuel base which allows very rapid energy conversion, this results in a rapid contraction speed. However, fast twitch activity is only efficient for a very short period, the waste by-products will eventually impede muscle function if allowed to concentrate. They are subdivided into two types:

1 FT I (Fast glycolytic – FG)
   • Their contractile properties are rapid.
   • They can function in the absence of oxygen.
   • They have larger glycogen stores than do ST fibres.
   • The circulatory network is not as dense so the removal of waste is less efficient.
2 FT II (Fast oxidative glycolytic – FOG)
   • These fibres display some characteristics of both previous groups ST and FT I.
   • They respond to exercise demands and build accordingly. Thus it is possible either to increase their ability to work in an anaerobic capacity increasing speed, or build their endurance abilities by working slowly against resistance.

FT types I and II are improved by fast work with reduced load.

To understand the likely evolutionary reasons for this muscle mix, it is essential to remember the requirements of both man and horse in their wild, natural states. The horse recruited fast twitch fibres in an explosive burst of energy which enabled it to run away from its predators, and then reduced speed, moving at a much slower pace as it continued to move away from the danger zone. Man recruited fast twitch fibres as he chased his prey and then recruited slow twitch as he either returned with his prize or walked sadly home.

Breed characteristics

As previously suggested. it is the feature of cross- or inter-breeding which creates one of the many problems when considering natural training, namely, what are the predominant characteristics of the muscles with which you are working?

Some breeds have a predominance of slow twitch fibres in their inherited genes and are therefore more suited to be trained for tasks which require stamina, for example in the Arabian, slow twitch or endurance muscle characteristics predominate.

The crossing of the Shire (slow twitch/endurance) to the TB (fast twitch/speed) is an attempt to achieve a good mix – the speed of the TB coupled to the endurance of the Shire. However, problems are still present when deciding on the appropriate the training regime. Which genetic inheritance is predominant in the muscle of this cross-bred horse?

Unfortunately, other than by carrying out muscle biopsy to identify the muscle composition, there is no way of knowing whether the result of cross-breeding, even with the animal looking like a TB, should be trained for endurance or speed-related sports and visa versa. Why does the offspring of the Shire mare, bred to a TB and looking like a Shire, simply fail to develop muscles as required? Of course, anything is possible, but the appropriate methods for muscle conditioning must be selected. Before purchase and however much you like the animal in question, it is always worthwhile standing back and deciding what you want to do with the horse. The old proverb 'you cannot make a silk purse out of a sow's ear' is relevant.

Further reading

Snow, D.H. & Vogel, C. *Equine Fitness*, David and Chalres, Newton Abbot, 1987

13 Anatomical Considerations

If the horse exists under natural conditions then over a period of time it will undergo skeletal and muscle development governed not just as a result of genetic factors but also secondary to the conditions supplied by varied terrain, the nutritional state of the individual animal and the fact that the horse will probably only rarely be required to move fast, and even then only for short periods of time.

If the feral horse becomes tired as a foal, it stops playing and running with its friends until it is ready, after a rest, to play again. When running free it does not suddenly meet a fence at the end of its paddock causing it to brake violently, which is detrimental to immature joints and particularly the hocks, it simply stops as it runs out of energy.

The valuable young Lipizzaners, destined for the Spanish Riding School in Vienna, are not kept in small paddocks. To avoid them hurting themselves they are turned away on the Alps for the first three years of their lives. When they begin formal training they are balanced, muscled and have very well-developed feet. The situation is similar in all feral horses.

Prepare slowly

To understand the importance of slow preparation consider the fact that in the horse approximately 206 individual bones are assembled to create the scaffold or frame. It is important also to understand that the frame must be held together which is primarily the job of ligaments aided by the muscles. Both of these tissues use the bones of the frame as a point of anchorage. Both tissues are carefully designed to exert maximum functional effect in the area over which they exert control.

The central scaffold or axial skeleton (see Fig. 13.1)

The axial components of the body frame are built around a central, multi-jointed rod – the vertebral column. They consist of the head, seven cervical vertebrae, or bones, of the neck, eighteen thoracic vertebrae which support the thorax or rib cage (so called because the ribs arise from the thoracic area of the vertebral column). From the thoracic cage the body frame goes from the loins, formed by the lumber vertebrae (usually six), to the pelvis, embracing the sacrum (five fused bones) between the ilial wings. The junction between sacrum and pelvic wings occurs at the two sacroiliac joints. The bones of the column end in those of the tail.

Within the main frame, the axial skeleton, are housed the abdominal contents, lungs, heart, reproductive organs, circulatory and nervous systems. The sum total of all bones

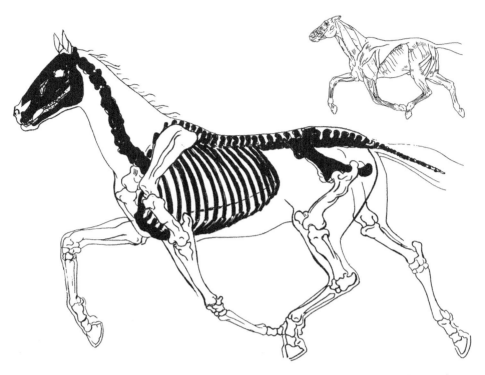

Fig. 13.1 Diagrammatic representation of the components of the axial skeleton in bold. Head, neck (cervical vertebrae), thorax (thoracic vertebrae, ribs and sternum), loins (lumbar vertebrae), pelvis, tail (caudal or coccygeal vertebrae).

and soft tissues when joined together, and the systems contained within, comprise the body mass.

Axial stability

As previously stated, movement of the limbs on the body mass requires a stable yet flexible axial frame. Consider the chassis, or frame, of a racing car, and think of the care with which mechanics check not only the tyres but also every nut and bolt holding the car together at each pit stop. An unstable chassis does not allow efficient wheel activity (limbs) or steering (balance). However, while stability is essential, total rigidity is counter productive, and shock absorption is essential (joints). This is due to the fact from an engineering point of view, that a totally rigid structure will eventually break.

Every structure, living or man made, must incorporate a controlled range of flexibility. Skyscrapers need to sway, a suspension bridge incorporates flexibility in its design and their construction is remarkably similar to the design of the horse's back.

It should be noted that neither horse nor rider is being helped under current legislation. The rider's natural body movement is severely constricted by rigid body protectors. The inability to move and thereby remain in balance with your horse is detrimental to both species.

In the horse, the construction of the thoracic portion of the axial skeleton or area behind the withers, usually described as 'the back', enjoys a natural, inbuilt stability due both to the shape of the eighteen individual vertebrae and the attached frame afforded by the ribs, but some flexibility is inherent in the design.

In order to get a three-dimensional picture of the thoracic portion of the body picture think of an upturned boat, the shape is similar to the thoracic cage. The rider sits astride the hull facing the bow of the boat, this representing the narrow front of the thoracic cage; the stern, behind the rider, is wider than the bow, this represents the width of the pelvis. The construction of a boat allows for very small movements within the frame; if it were totally rigid then the structure would break up under stress. The thoracic cage is similar and, contrary to general belief, the design ensures very little movement.

Leverage

A leverage system, supplied by the four limbs, is attached to the central mass – the front limbs to the thoracic cage, the hind limbs to the pelvis.

The limbs suspend and balance the central mass, holding it off the ground, supporting the huge weight and resisting the downward pull of gravitational forces. The limbs are also designed and are able, by virtue of muscle and tendon activity, to achieve a series of variable levers. These levers use muscle energy to become active, supply the power required to move the body over ground, or, if the horse is required to jump fences, upward into the air.

Consider the fact that this massive weight, sometimes as great as 0.75 tonne or more, achieves the air-borne phase in all gaits, as well as when jumping, as the result of the power exerted by one hind limb, and that a single front limb bears the strain when connection with the ground occurs on landing.

It must be recognised that building the stability of the frame or axial skeleton is essential for performance. Stability is achieved partially by architectural design but is aided by muscle arrangement in association with ligaments. The deep muscles holding the frame, the multi-bone structure, together are described as postural muscles. The way they are arranged and the fibre pattern are designed to achieve stability rather than movement. These muscles build naturally in early training if the body is not subjected to rider weight.

Unfortunately, rather as the human back has areas of weakness or the tendency to be unstable in certain areas, so does that of the horse. The demands of modern competition and, for many horses, a sedentary lifestyle contribute to unacceptable muscular skeletal stress in the vulnerable areas.

Two of the weakest areas in the axial skeleton of the horse are:

- the junction between the last neck or cervical vertebra, C7, and the first of the eighteen vertebrae forming the central 'rod' of the thoracic cage, T1.
- the junction described as L6/S1, sited between the last, or sixth, lumbar vertebra (loin area) and the first of the five, fused vertebrae, forming the sacrum, which is attached, as previously described, to the ilial wings of the pelvis.

C7, T1 (see Fig. 13.2)

The seventh cervical or last neck vertebra, C7, meets T1, the first thoracic or chest vertebra, deep between the two shoulder blades, the scapulae. During pure forward movement at walk, it is at this joint that the 'up and down' movements of neck and head on

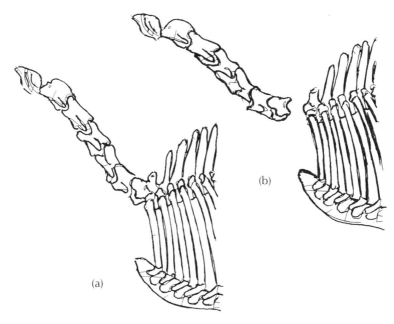

Fig. 13.2 A weak junction – last neck vertebra C7 to the thoracic cage T1. (a) the seventh cervical vertebra joins the thoracic cage at T1. (b) the neck vertebrae detached from the thorax. All movements of head and neck on the body mass occur at this junction.

the body mass, occur, 'head nodding' being a peculiar characteristic of the walk. This junction takes the strain of all neck movements and is also subjected to the weight of head, despite the fact that the cervical vertebrae are suspended from a very important ligament, the nuchal ligament. Due to the arrangement of the long back muscles, stability of the entire back is inter-related with this area.

L6, S1

The hind legs are attached to the pelvis through the hip joints, a bone union, to ensure stability for the powerful thrust achieved by the massive hind quarter musculature. The range of movement to achieve the thrusting power developed by the hind limbs requires adaptations in the architectural shape of both the body, and most importantly the posterior spine, of the last lumbar vertebra, L6, and also of the first of the five fused sacral vertebrae, S1; these are obvious when a skeletal specimen is viewed (see Fig. 13.3).

At this junction, the articulating surfaces between the bodies of the vertebrae have flattened, the posterior spine of L6 is angled forward or cranially, while the spine of S1 is angled backward or caudally. This design and the arrangement of the local musculature enables a small amount of flexion and extension at this very important junction which is required to enable the horse to make full use of the power in the hind legs and quarters. The movement at the junction L6/S1 enables the horse to take the hind leg further forward under the body mass than if the area were fixed, then plant the foot and initiate thrust by limb extension in order to push the entire body mass over the previously planted fore leg. Horses weak in this area do not enjoy the thrust power of those horses which are adequately muscled in their loins.

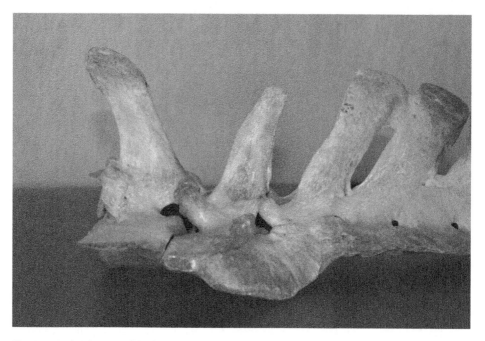

Fig. 13.3 Left side view of the lumbar sacral junction, L6/S1. Note the angles of the posterior spines, L6 (left of figure) angles forward toward the head, S1 (adjacent) angles back towards the tail.

Nuchal ligament

In most horses the poll, the top of the skull, is positioned slightly higher than the highest point of the withers. The head is attached to the body through articulation with the first neck vertebrae or *atlas*. Movement between these two structures is flexion and extension, or, nose poked forward, nose tucked in – an important point when assessing break over. The atlas articulates with the second neck vertebra or *axis*, at this junction rotation or side turning of the head is possible, nose tilted to the left or the right, these very specific movements rely on small local muscles. Full neck usage should incorporate these two localised movements, particularly as head position is concerned with balance, limb co-ordination and the position of the back. Break over, or flexion, which occurs only at the atlanto-occipital joint is incorrect and, as will become clear later in the text, the horse's back will suffer.

The bones of the neck from the axis are arranged in a curve resembling an inverted, flattened 'S'. This structure is secured by numerous ligaments. Of these, the most important ligament in the horse's body is the nuchal ligament which rises from the top of the skull, the area known as the poll, or in anatomical terms, the external occipital protuberance. The nuchal ligament is described in two parts. The lamella section of the circular elastic ligament first bridges the gap created by the arrangement of the neck vertebrae between the poll and the highest point of the withers. This landmark, the tip of the longest of the thoracic spines, is usually T4. At the position of T4, the ligament widens and is attached in the wither area both to the tips and sides of the thoracic spines forming the wither contour. Then, just behind the withers the structure narrows and flattens to

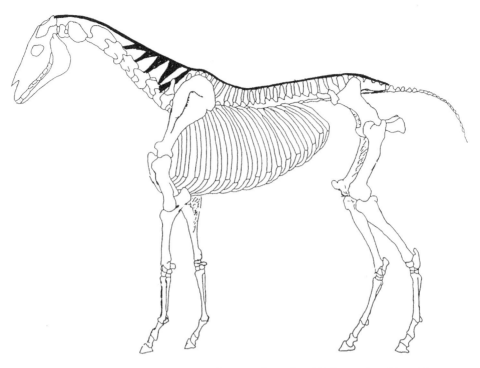

Fig. 13.4 Nuchal ligament bridging the gap between the poll and highest point of the withers, continuing, renamed as the supraspinous ligament, to the sacrum.

continue, centrally placed, along the entire length of the back to the sacrum. It moulds directly with the tissue comprising the tips of each vertebral spine and their interspinous ligaments. From withers to sacrum, the nuchal ligament is renamed, becoming the supraspinous ligament.

After the lamella section has passed above the atlas and axis with no connection to either bone, the funicular portion of the ligament forms, fibres arise from the under, or ventral, aspect of the lamella section, creating a fan-like arrangement of fibrous bands. These fibrous bands pass down and forward, filling the gap created by the curve of the 'S' and lock, at their distal ends, onto the remaining five cervical vertebrae and by so doing suspend the individual bones. This fan of fibres also creates an area within the central neck for muscle anchorage (see Fig. 13.4).

The bone arrangement of the 'S' shape is very mobile and changes continually as the horse moves head and neck. These changes may either reduce or increase tension throughout the entire ligament structure *involving and including* the section lying along the centre of the back.

The variations in tension throughout the entire structure – the lamella, funicular and supraspinous portions – created by head position, affect suspension throughout the entire central rod of the axial skeleton, the vertebral column.

It is very important for the rider to understand correct 'break over'. This involves the slight repositioning of all the neck vertebrae, *not* just flexion at the atlanto-occipital joint, which results in the horse being 'behind the bit'. In this situation there is minimal increase in the generalised support of the back, and the horse, although bent in the neck,

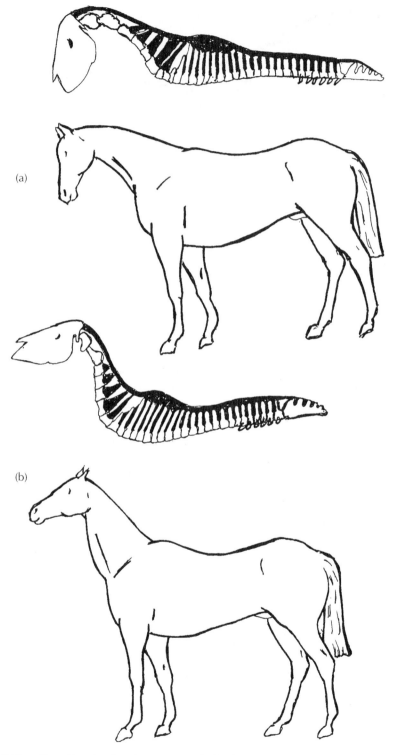

Fig. 13.5 The effect of head and neck position on the back. (a) even break over achieves a traction effect helping to suspend or lift the back. (b) high head carriage, or going above the bit, reduces traction with a resultant hollow back.

still has a hollow back. This lack of support also occurs with a high head carriage, reduced tension throughout the ligaments which leads to poor back suspension. Result – a hollow back (see Fig. 13.5).

Even break over achieves increased traction from poll to sacrum, with subsequent, improved back suspension. The ligaments assist the muscles of the back to stabilise and lift the structure enabling the horse to carry a rider, and also to move the limbs efficiently in response to rider requirement.

All riders and trainers should appreciate that it is impossible to divorce the neck section of the vertebral column from the thoracic and lumbar sections. The 'back' is usually mistakenly considered to only be the area on which the rider sits.

Muscle support of the axial skeleton

The neck musculature fills the area between the nuchal ligament and cervical vertebrae. The fibre direction of the individual muscles is arranged according to function. Muscles are also sited on the underside of the neck vertebrae, unlike the thoracic area, where the muscles are sited *only* on the upper aspect of the ribs and along the sides of the spines of the vertebrae.

Just as the long muscles of the back run forward into the neck area, using cervical vertebrae as their anchorage point, so some of the muscles of the neck pass backwards to anchor on the ribs. This arrangement, and therefore attention paid to building these muscles, is very important to ensure a fully functional, well-supported junction of neck to body mass. Poor functional development of the muscle mass at the base of the neck interferes with the ability of the neck not only to support the back but, as the horse uses its head and neck to balance, this essential feature is also compromised.

In the loins, a very important muscle group gives support on the *under or ventral surface* of the vertebrae. Originating within the pelvis, the fibres of the muscle named ileo psoas pass forward beneath the sacroiliac joint (also supporting the area) and end attached beneath the lateral projections of the lumbar vertebrae.

The arrangement of the abdominal musculature (abdominal tunic) is primarily one of restraint rather than of movement, for the abdominal contents must be retained within the body mass. While the muscles do become involved in the movement of the pelvis on the last lumbar vertebra (lumbo-sacral joint), the abdominal muscles are not the main supporting groups of the back as is often commonly supposed. When the hind limb is brought under the body mass the abdominals assist by drawing the lower part of the pelvis forward towards their anchorage area, the thoracic cage. This action assists ileo psoas to achieve the necessary flexion at the lumbo-sacral joint and so allow the hind limb to move as far forward under the body as the conformation of the horse and/or the movement to be executed requires. At the conclusion of lumbo-sacral joint flexion, abdominal muscle action momentarily helps to lift the back. However, at the moment when the hind limb support phase occurs, the centre of gravity must shift, both to allow diaphragmatic respiration and to enable the horse to remain in balance. This would not be possible if there were undue tension in the abdominal tunic so the muscles relax. If the abdominal muscles were the main supporting group of the back this relaxation would be catastrophic.

The traction effect (see Fig. 13.5), created throughout the nuchal and supraspinous ligaments, secondary to the position of head and neck, and the long back muscles determine back position (see Fig. 13.6).

In the un-ridden horse, the muscle/ligament arrangement of the back is very energy efficient, with the horse able to position the head and neck to suit its requirements;

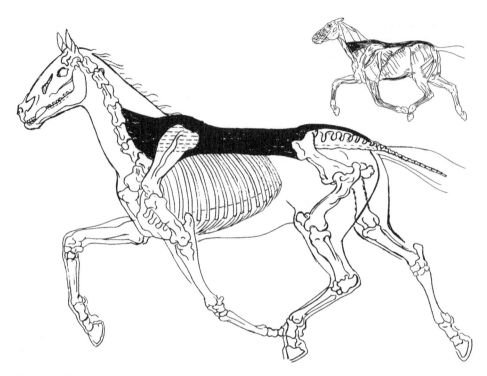

Fig. 13.6 The muscles of the back interweave and form a long, uninterrupted chain, stretching from neck to pelvis.

lowering the head when going uphill lifts the back, enabling hind limb activity to become the priority, rather than wasting energy unnecessarily through having to hold the back in position. Riding naturally suggests, if the slope is very steep the rider should get off and walk.

14 Appendicular Skeleton – The Levers

The levers are composed of a series of single bones for the most part balanced one upon another, and in some joints, for example at the elbow, interlocking (see Fig. 14.1).

The front limbs (see Fig. 14.2)

These are the predominantly weight-bearing structures in the horse, taking 60% of the body weight, but unlike the hind limbs, which enjoy a bone attachment for stability, they are not joined to the axial frame other than by muscles.

The muscles of attachment have a quadruple role:

- attaching the fore limbs to the thoracic cage;
- stabilising the fore limbs;
- providing, in association with the long back muscles, a suspension and stabilising mechanism for the front section of the thoracic cage – the thoracic sling;
- assisting in the attachment of head and neck to the thoracic cage and thus to the body mass.

It follows that if the muscle groups, particularly those spanning the junction between the base of neck and thoracic cage, are poorly developed, then the underlying area of the thoracic cage, to which the front limbs attach, will be unstable. Some of these important muscles involved in stability of the area are active, working and increasing their functional capability, as the head nods at walk. *Too often this naturally endowed movement is restricted by side reins when a horse is worked from the ground, this is totally counter-productive.*

The necessity for stability at the front, or cranial, end of the thoracic cage appears least understood and is poorly addressed in most training programmes, when emphasis is usually directed primarily at hock engagement and outline. Neither of these require-ments can be achieved until the weight-bearing fore limbs, between which the thoracic cage is suspended, are fully secure, both in the development of their individual stay sys-tems and their attachment to the body mass.

Because the horse possesses a subconscious, or in-built, survival programme, it instinctively realises it cannot achieve a long stride if the structure to which the fore limbs attach lacks stability. Thus, inadequate underlying support will not allow the weight-bearing fore limb to extend fully. Not only does this result in a shortened stride in front, but there will also be a compensatory reduction of hind limb stride length.

Instinct tells the horse not to use a full stride from behind as the front leg is in the way and the toe of the hind limb is in danger of clipping and damaging the back of the fore limb. This change of gait, prompted by survival instincts, results in the horse tending to go up and down on the spot rather than covering ground.

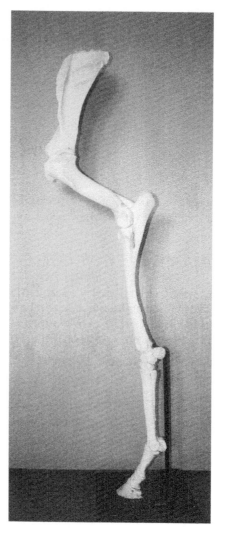

Fig. 14.1 Lateral view of the left front limb. The bones are, for the most part, balanced one upon another. Only at the elbow do the bones interlock.

The hind limbs

The hind limbs are the horse's power levers. They carry around 40% of the body weight and, unlike the fore limbs, gain stability and strength via a bone attachment to the axial skeleton (see Fig. 14.3). The femur is the first bone of the hind limb lever, with the hip joint the area of attachment. Design has sited a ligament inside the hip joint, the structure running from the head of the femur to the pelvis. This supplies the stability necessary for the hind limb to achieve its functional requirements, creating the power to propel the body mass over the planted fore limb at all speeds, or upwards, when jumping.

The hind limb levers not only differ in their mechanism of attachment from the fore limbs, but also because the stifle joint of the hind limb possesses a unique feature – the ability, by manipulation, of one of the patella tendons to lock the joint. One totally stable limb allows the horse to doze in the standing position.

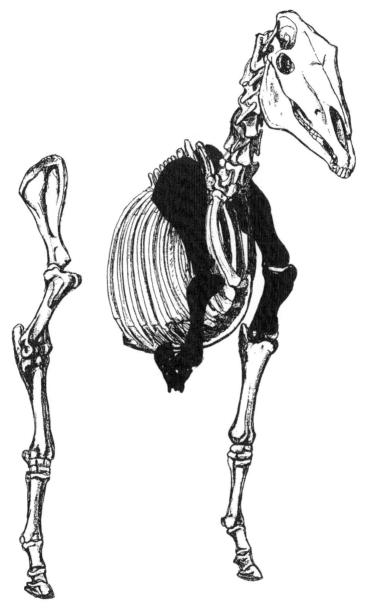

Fig. 14.2 The front limbs are attached to the thoracic cage by muscles. In the diagram, the right front limb is shown detached, the blocked out area on the thoracic cage indicates the position of attachment.

This is yet another survival feature of the horse. Should danger threaten if the horse were lying on the ground resting, it would takes longer for it to rise onto its feet. Unlocking a fixed joint enables the animal to run instantly if it is already standing.

The massive muscles of the hind quarter mass and those of the flank are arranged for pendulum-type movements of the limbs, incorporating positioning and thrust. The hind quarters constitute the movement powerhouse, using the leverage of the hind limb to direct the power generated in order to catapult the body mass forwards, upwards or to the side.

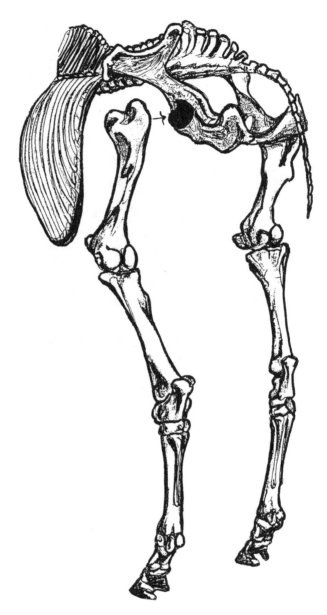

Fig. 14.3 The hind limbs are joined to the pelvis by an internal ligament within the hip joint. This joint creates a bone union between the leg and body mass. In the diagram, the left hind limb is shown detached. The small, blocked out area on the pelvis indicates the site where the head of the femur joints to the body mass.

The thrust of the hind limbs is alternate. The force generated is transmitted through the hip joint to the pelvic wing of the same side, the force then passes through the junction between pelvis and sacrum (see Fig. 14.4), the minute sacroiliac joint, and is transmitted to the vertebral column. The result of this is movement of the entire body mass in the direction required.

To ensure economy of effort, the pelvis must be stable when subjected to one-sided force. This requires activity in the loin muscles acting on the opposite pelvic wing. Poor devel-

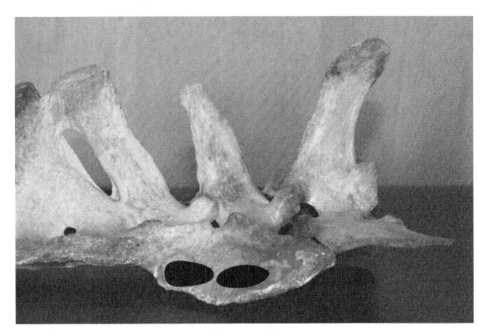

Fig. 14.4 The right side of the sacrum. The blocked-out area indicates the tiny lower, or sacral, surface of the sacroiliac joint. The opposite surface is formed by an area of identical size on the underside of the ilial wing.

opment of the musculature in the loins creates an unstable area and thrust power will not be distributed correctly. Similarly, an imbalance between left and right loin musculature will also affect drive-force distribution. Any imbalance of force, applied to any structure, results in uneven stresses. To the discerning reader it should be obvious that if the forces transmitted by hind limb thrust are out of balance for whatever reason, then the sacroiliac joints and the loins, including the vertebral column, must be affected (see Fig. 14.5).

The sacroiliac joint is subjected to a shearing force in the loins due to its design. A rotational force results if an imbalance between right and left thrust occurs which leads to back discomfort after exercise.

Balance of power between left and right hind limbs reduces risk in the natural horse, and as the back is not required to carry weight, problems are rare.

The thrust power from a single hind leg is transmitted through the hip joint to the sacroiliac joint, thence via the lumbo-sacral joint to the vertebral column. The effect of this is to propel the entire body mass over the supporting front leg when jumping, to propel the body upwards. In Fig. 14.5, the shoulder of the supporting leg, the left front, is slightly advanced. The pelvis is stabilised by the loin muscles on the opposite side to the working hind leg.

Lateral movement

Besides moving the body mass forwards, backwards and upwards, the four limb levers are also able to move the body sideways. To achieve what riders call 'lateral movements', the limbs must use muscle groups positioned and designed to achieve limb stability during movement, rather than to initiate movement, these groups are known as adductors and abductors.

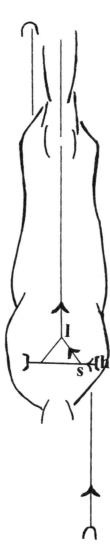

Fig. 14.5 Diagram of the outline of a horse from above, to demonstrate the effect of the thrust power of a hind leg. The right hind is the working leg. h) hip joint, s) sacroiliac joint, l) lumbo-sacral joint.

The thrust power from a single hind leg is transmitted through the hip joint to the sacroiliac joint, thence via the lumbo-sacral joint to the vertebral column. The effect of this is to propel the entire body mass over the supporting front leg when jumping, to propel the body upwards. In the diagram, the shoulder of the supporting leg, the left front, is slightly advanced. The pelvis is stabilised by the loin muscles on the opposite side to the working hind leg.

During forwards or backwards movement of the limbs, these groups function to ensure that individual limbs do not fall inwards, adduction, or outward, abduction (see Figs. 14.6 and 14.7).

Consider the pattern of movement of the front limb. Scapula and humerus are directly attached to the thoracic cage, the solid frame of the cage prevents the bones moving inwards and muscle attachment holds them to the cage preventing them from moving outwards away from the body mass. The remaining components of the limb present as a jointed rod held together by the stay system. (See Fig. 14.8.)

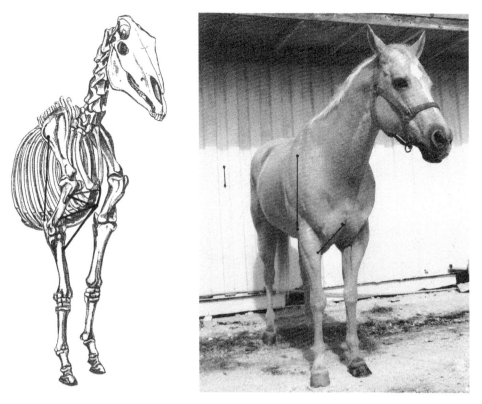

Fig. 14.6 The position of the ad- and abductor muscles of the right fore limb. The adductor muscles form the masses easily identified between the front legs. Muscles running from elbow to scapula on the lateral aspect of the shoulder act, when required, as abductors.

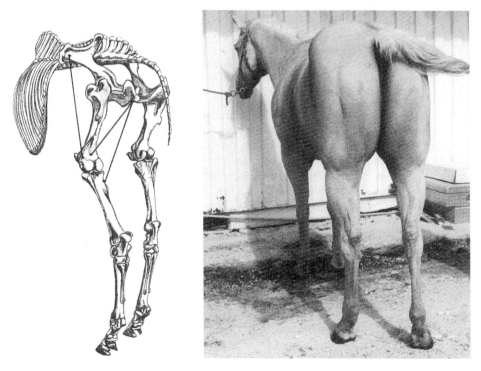

Fig. 14.7 The position of the ad- and abductor muscles of the left hind limb. The adductor muscles form the masses between the hind limbs. Muscles running from pelvis to femur on the flank, act as abductors when required.

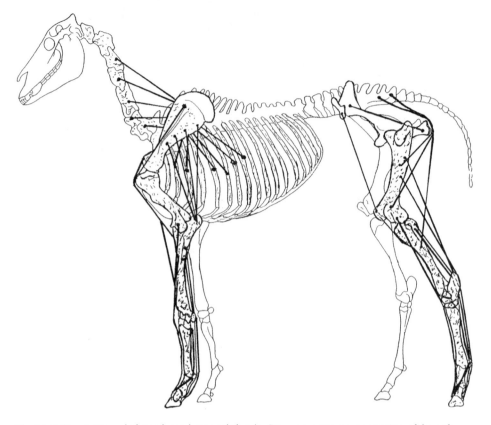

Fig. 14.8 Stay system, skeleton lateral aspect left side. Diagrammatic representation of the soft tissue arrangement comprising the stay system. The soft tissue structures sited on the front and back of the limbs maintain a balanced equilibrium of force between themselves to counteract gravity and retain the position of the individual bones forming the limbs.

As the limb advances, the foot meets the ground, straight in front of the body mass, following the airborne phase of movement. The foot, and the jointed rod, spanning the gap between ground and thoracic cage, needs to remain stable with the foot the point of balance enabling the body mass to move forwards. The adductor muscles prevent the rod falling outwards, the abductor muscles prevent the rod falling inwards.

The need to consider these groups when training the horse is often not understood. For limb stability in early education and later for trouble-free lateral movements and also for also circling, attention to the development of, and balance between, ab- and adductor groups cannot be emphasised too strongly. (With the concept of balance, we are back to Chinese philosophy!)

The stay system (see Fig. 14.8)

The limbs, described in anatomical terms as the appendicular skeleton, consist in the main of single, individual bones balancing one upon or against another. Muscles, ligaments and tendons are arranged to ensure that the bones remain or 'stay' correctly positioned, the design requiring minimal muscle effort and so conserving energy.

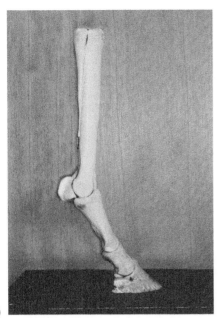
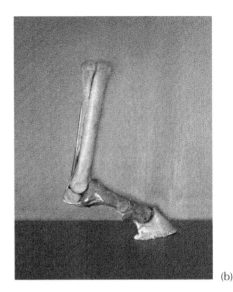

(a)   (b)

Fig. 14.9 a&b (a) Normally, the sesamoid bones sited behind the fetlock joint bear no weight. (b) The sesamoid bones repositioned to support the full body weight momentarily as at fast paces the pastern lies parallel to the ground.

The design configuration enables the soft tissue components of the 'stay system' to work with adjacent muscle groups, assisting in conversion of the standing bone arrangement to the levers required to achieve body mass movement. At the conclusion of activity the system resumes maintenance of the standing position.

There are no muscles in the lower or distal part of the limbs. This results in the distal portion, the segments from knee and hock to ground, in both front and hind limbs, becoming the most vulnerable areas in the horse.

The bone arrangement is such that collapse of a limb would tend to be backwards. Support to avoid collapse at fetlock and pastern joints is provided by constant activity within the suspensory ligament aided by the tendons of the superficial and deep flexor muscles. On the front of each limb one tendon, the common digital extensor tendon, provides the necessary counter-traction force. The amazing tensile strength of these structures, particularly of the suspensory ligament, is to a degree illustrated by the fact that at full gallop the pastern of the weight-bearing limb lies parallel to the ground. This opens the fetlock joint to such a degree that normal bone connection between the cannon and pastern bone is lost. Momentarily, the only component available to take the full weight of the horse is provided by the suspensory ligament using the two sesamoid bones suspended within its structure (see Fig. 14.9 a&b).

Normally, the sesamoid bones are sited just behind the fetlock joints, enclosed in the tissue of the suspensory ligament, one towards the inner, the other towards the outer aspect. As pastern-to-ground angle changes, the suspensory ligament is pulled downwards and the bones reposition, lying below as opposed to behind, the distal end of the cannon bone. Arranged thus, they function in association with traction supplied by the suspensory ligament and the tendons of the superficial and deep digital flexors, to support the full body weight passing down through the limb preventing the distal end of the cannon bone making contact with the ground.

Understanding activity

Muscles build and adapt in response to functional demand to achieve improved capability. Improved capability above and beyond that needed for natural living necessitates the implementation of resistance.

Resistance, when considered as an adjunct to training muscle, involves creating tasks which require muscles to work over and above their current known capability. For horses living in a domesticated situation, this requires designing activities which will involve preselected sets of muscles. The activities selected will demand extra work for the targeted groups. Today's domestic horse tends to be trained on a 'safe', man-designed surface, with little or no exposure in many cases to any variation. It should come as no surprise that a horse trained on one type of surface and then asked to compete on another will not move as expected. The body is suddenly and unexpectedly exposed to signals never before experienced, and while the well-schooled animal will do its best to comply with rider command, overall performance will suffer.

The Golden Horse Shoe Ride on Exmoor provides an annual example to illustrate the necessity for variation. Horses need time to become moor wise, heather is hard work, the ground surface undulating and uneven, and both take their toll. Many animals are withdrawn from the ride at the first check point because they are exhausted despite having previously completed 100 mile tracks over flat country without any problems.

In a natural environment the horse builds the muscles of both axial and appendicular skeleton as it moves during daily life. In a feral state the horse enjoys endless changes in body position, is exposed to varied terrain, long distances, slopes, varied ground conditions, it also changes gait depending on herd behaviour. It is for these reasons – continued exposure to a variety of situations, allowing development over time, with only short periods of concentrated effort – that feral horses once tamed are found to be well muscled, balanced and move with confidence, carrying riders easily.

The desert-raised Arabian, the Mongolian horse of the steppes, horses that work cattle in Australia and the Argentine and the feral horses of north America, all stabilise their frames as the result of living in way that is as nearly natural as that enjoyed by the original wild species. In the UK there is a term 'as sure footed as a mountain pony'. This does not refer to balance alone, for balance and performance are secondary to axial frame stability, which is something that can only be provided by muscle support. The other, old terminology used to describe a well-balanced, successful horse stated that 'whatever happens he always finds a fifth leg'.

Early training should concentrate on building a stable frame. This requires consideration of the bone scaffold and the postural muscles functioning to hold the frame together before anything else. There is little point in implementing any training routine designed to strengthen muscle if the frame, on which the muscles rely for anchorage, cannot resist the stresses created by their activity. Muscle training for eventual ridden work follows on from frame stability.

The skeletal frame, beginning as cartilage *in utero*, is almost completely calcified by the time of birth. However, the bones continue to develop for several years, the time of greatest activity being during the first few years of life. Unfortunately, no exact timescale for completion of growth can be given, many owners have bought a five-year-old, which to their amazement, or in the case of show animals, horror, have grown when given a nutritious diet.

No body tissue is inert, tissues respond and remodel according to the stresses to which they are subjected. In common with all other tissues, bone is continuously repairing and remodelling in response to the stresses to which it is subjected and this continues throughout the life of the animal.

The natural horse is exposed to a variety of ground surfaces, each delivering a different resonance or impaction force at the point of contact. The shock waves experienced on impact are partially dissipated within the foot, but are also transmitted to the bones following hoof–ground contact. The resonance experienced is also subject to a wide range of variation, not only from the type of surface but also from that speed of contact, foot-to-ground angle, the slope of the ground and whether it is a slippage or holding-type ground. All these features create a different resonance and each stimulates bone. The response to stimulation results in the body remodelling the internal structural architecture in a manner, in the case of bone, to prepare against possible damage or catastrophic break down under future stress.

Of course, the resonance experienced by bone is also influenced by shoes. Metal creates its own resonance on meeting a surface. In the shod animal, poor foot balance and the type of shoe must always be considered. Is the horse landing medially stressing the medial splint bone with possible resultant splint development?

There is a tendency in the natural approach to let the horses go barefoot. It will take time for the bone to adapt to a new resonance following removal of shoes from a previously shod horse. Neither does no shoe mean no trimming. Poorly shaped feet, even though bare, will not dissipate the resonance created by ground contact efficiently and may well create, rather than reduce, skeletal stresses. Over time, the barefoot horse will, if in receipt of appropriate nutrients, develop a thicker sole and a resilient hoof wall which will enable the animal to remain unshod and will assist to a degree in resonance dissipation.

While the natural horse prepares in its own 'gym', the domestic animal tends to be prepared in an arena with a 'safe' surface. Early work for a horse was originally done in long reins, the horses driven at walk, from the ground. They were *walked* on a variety of surfaces, over tarmac, down lanes, through woods, across grass and plough, often for at least the first three months of formal education. This regime not only subjected the skeleton to variation, involved a requirement for good self-carriage and natural balance, but also activated the postural muscles, whose function is to create a stable frame prior to the addition of rider weight.

In their later life, after a holiday break, horses used to be subjected to at least six to eight weeks walking on the roads when preparation began. 'Road work' was considered to strengthen their legs. However, this suggestion is too much of a generalisation, 'legs' should be interpreted as encompassing all the structures: bone, ligaments and tendons. The bone structure is certainly subjected to stimulation by road work, the bones of the legs are of huge importance and as previously discussed it is essential to prepare the skeletal frame.

Blyth Tait, event rider and Olympic gold medallist, had his horses walked in hand, daily for an hour or more, for a minimum of four to six weeks after their short autumn break, before they started pre-season training.

Unfortunately, due to modern traffic conditions, road work is no longer safe or advisable in many areas, but dry, firm ground in a large field is useful; tracks, paths over heath or moor if available and firm sand, all offer essential resonance variety.

There is a second important reason for variety of surface usage. Neural receptors in the feet are stimulated as the foot meets the ground. Known as proprioceptors, their activity is essential for the body mass to function efficiently and most importantly they are involved in balance. These important neural receptors rely for stimulation and education on exposure to as many variations in footage as possible.

In his rehabilitation programme, Jean Marie Denoix DVM uses a long walk way broken down into sections; each section floored with different components – fine gravel, coarse gravel, cinders, rubber, pebbles. Horses are walked up and down the track to stimulate their proprioceptive input.

A noted yard in the UK has built a walker with the floor made from smooth pebbles of varying sizes. They feel the balance ability of the horses walked over this surface to be vastly improved. The stables of domestic horses used to be made of cobbles. Did our forebears recognise something we have missed?

15 Training

A distinguished pedigree or parentage is no guarantee of success. No athlete will reach their full potential without years of diligent help (training) to optimise and develop their skills. In the horse, unlike the human, the programme of all the skills necessary for living and survival is present in the brain at birth. As riders or trainers we use the horse brain's preloaded or inherent skills, to teach the horse to react in a specific manner, in response to delivered signals. Liken the equine brain to a computer. When purchased all the basic information for function is preloaded, you, as the computer operator, expand on the installed programmes. Training the horse could be regarded as a similar activity. By understanding the preloaded programme you can build and improve on information already stored.

Of course, using a computer requires the understanding and operation of the keyboard. Your manipulation of the keyboard generates the appropriate electronic signals to ensure the 'brain' of the computer (hard drive) responds to your wishes. What is the keyboard in the horse? How are the signals given?

It is by using reflex areas, described earlier in this text, that we communicate with the horse, using the signals we term 'aids'. Some of these reflex areas are sited in the back but predominately they are on the horse's side, described by Bruce Davidson, one-time Olympic rider for the USA and gold medallist, as the magic triangle. The horse responds through its inbuilt, complex reflex chain of neural responses, learning to lift the back, strike off on a selected leg and change legs in response to the 'aids'. The reaction occurs as a movement or series of movements, which in the wild would be a *natural* reaction to ensure survival. The signals, in a simplistic form, work as follows. Something presses against your side, the *reaction* is to step sideways to avoid contact; or there may be a subtle shift of rider weight including side contact, the *reaction* is to retain balance by changing the leading leg, and so on.

Eventually, when a signal is given, the horse responds by moving, turning, halting, changing direction, changing gait or changing legs. The rider must choose a separate signal for each movement. Confusion arises if the horse is given an incorrect or indecisive signal. Its brain does not know how to react and the horse fails to produce the movement required by the rider. Clarity and exact repetition of command are essential; punishment causes resentment.

As you manipulate the brain responses, you can, over a period of time, build on the programmed reactions to expand capability. This can only happen slowly. First request a simple response, in very early training, for example, when halted get the horse to stand square. Gradually over a period of time, and by using exact repetition of the signal or command used to achieve a square halt, the brain will install the information, 'when I halt I must stand square' and the response will then become automatic.

Only if the signals are repeated often enough will the horse's brain log them and it will eventually respond by performing the movement that it has learnt to be the correct, required response. Some horses learn faster than others, some have an apparent in-built capacity to perform tasks others find difficult. To achieve your goals it cannot be too strongly emphasised that schooling or teaching requires care and *most importantly time*.

Over a period of time, as rider and horse both come to understand and trust one another, response to the aids becomes an instinctive reaction in the movement area of the brain. Then, and only then, do the rider aids become so subtle that the horse appears to be working alone and yet he is in complete harmony with the rider.

The author has watched a number of riders, including Linda Tellington Jones, ride a complete dressage test with no bridle. Natural horsemen remember that you ride your horse by educating your seat and lower leg, not through the reins and possibly an associated bit.

As previously suggested, to become a horseman, natural or otherwise, requires the enhancement of rider reactions. Through contact the rider should not only be able to tell the horse what they, the rider require, but of equal importance, read the horse through their own legs, seat and hands. The following are some useful things to note:

- Has the back lifted? Does it feel soft?
- What is the state of balance?
- Does the horse feel tired or full of energy?
- Is it working through from behind?
- Is it heavy in front?
- Is the feel equal on both diagonals?
- Which canter lead is being used?
- Does the horse go disunited after a change of leg?

Prior to current regulations regarding safety, riding bareback was a superb learning activity. Treeless, close-contact saddles could be considered by riders hoping to hone their communication skills.

The domestic horse

Consider the requirements for athletic performance, for even with a natural approach the horse is destined to carry a rider. What is the best approach to educate a horse as naturally as possible under domestic conditions? If you do not wish to use an expert and want to bring on a young horse or improve an older animal, particularly if a change of discipline is involved, remember the feral horse and recreate, as nearly as possible, a routine of muscle building which enables the horse to build naturally.

Which features should help to ensure that the horse accepts, and eventually even enjoys an inter-relationship with man, including being ridden?

Fear is the first sense to address and consider. Mentally, the horse must become relaxed in the presence of man and also when exposed to new situations. This phase of training must *never be hurried*. Always give the horse *time* to appreciate that a new situation need not be harmful or dangerous. Attempting to educate an apprehensive horse is not only difficult but also unproductive for both man and horse.

Return to consideration of the importance of appreciating the inter-linkage between body systems. Mental apprehension is a neural response linked to inherent, instinctive behaviour where the mental state is triggered by messages passing via the autonomic nervous system. The peripheral neural system, controlling muscle, interlinks with the autonomic system responsible for registering a feeling of apprehension. Due to system interlinkage, the signal 'danger get ready to fight or flee', results in muscle tension, and so in this case muscle tension is secondary to apprehension. In the natural state, muscles may need to be on the alert, ready to enable the animal to flee, but when educating muscle, tension interferes with movement and every aspect of training.

It is *inadvisable to give treats* when the horse accepts a new situation as this can encourage unwanted behavioural patterns which you do not need. *Never forget* that all your actions are being logged into the computer – the horse's brain. Treats could be considered as a virus that pops up when least needed. At the end of a long day, you and the horse are tired. *You*: 'Come on into the trailer, let's get home.' *Horse*: 'Where is my carrot? I never get into that thing without a carrot.' No carrots to be had. Result: stalemate.

When using natural horsemanship, make use of horse behaviour – bonding, security, following acceptance of a situation, results within the herd, in self or allogrooming (see Fig. 15.1). Find the favourite spot on the neck and scratch it.

If it is programmed in, this method of reassurance will also help when the horse is mounted. By stimulating an installed programme, scratching the neck, you key into an installed brain response and persuade the horse to overcome a temporary, fear-induced attitude.

The brain sequence you keyed into ran roughly as follows – fear, tension, then, gradual acceptance of the experience/situation/task, 'it does not seem harmful'. The acceptance time period may include snorting, tail lifting, neck stretched to sniff, a step backward, pulling away, then via the natural, neural-induced acceptance path, reassurance. These principles are those so ably adapted by Monty Roberts and his team. It is

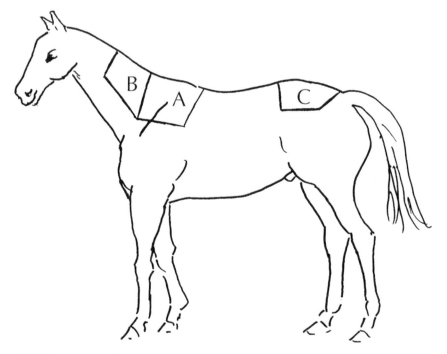

Fig. 15.1 Diagrammatic sketch of the left side of a horse showing the areas of self, or allogrooming. A: withers (first preference); B: mid neck (second preference); C: croup or top of hind quarter mass (third preference). Allogrooming is considered to subdue aggression, to encourage bonding and for cleaning.

worth repeating here that horse mastership cannot all be learned from a book. Go to joining-up demonstrations, watch, learn then implement.

Physical requirements

Which physical requirements should the rider aim for to ensure the horse becomes responsive, safe, educated and a pleasure to ride?

- *Straightness*: the horse should first learn to move straight. It is easier for the horse to stay in balance when moving straight, this is what nature intended.
  Crookedness is not always the fault of the horse, a rider sitting with their weight predominantly to one side results in the horse readjusting its body mass and as a result becoming crooked. Uneven contact through the rein will result in the horse turning the head toward the heavier hand, balance is compromised and results in crookedness.
- *Balance*: the horse should learn to be in balance which requires rhythm. Once this has been achieved with the horse riderless, it then has to be relearned by the horse as it accustoms itself to supporting weight on its back and has to modify the use of the muscles supporting neck and back.
- *Suppleness*: movement requirements should aim for easy, relaxed activity. This is often described as the horse being supple, but suppleness is actually secondary to muscle preparation. If muscles are prepared in a manner which results in good support of and control over the joints of the body, the horse instinctively realises that an increased range of joint movement can be performed safely. Well-prepared/toned muscles act like beautifully tempered springs.
- *Collection*: gradually, light contact will achieve collection. This occurs as the power generated by muscle becomes subtly contained and it is necessary in order to create impulsion.
- *Impulsion*: impulsion follows collection and could be described as having harnessed the power of the horse to achieve energetic movement.

None of these features can be achieved by rushing the first training, when changing from one discipline to another or retraining whatever the reason. All require at least a year, and preferably two, using very basic work.

Aims of natural training

The aims of natural training could embrace the following concepts:

(a) To appreciate that because of inbuilt responses which have developed due to the necessity for *herd safety*, the horse *expects* to learn *obedience*.
(b) To recreate as nearly as possible a natural living situation for the horse.
(c) To provide companionship, preferably equine.
(d) To allow time for interaction and musculo-skeletal preparation.
(e) To understand that each horse has a natural carriage peculiar to its conformation.
(f) To first teach the horse to go straight at all paces.
(g) To appreciate that for a horse to perform a circle requires a complicated and difficult set of movement patterns and muscle co-ordination.
(h) To build the musculo-skeletal systems as nature intended, using natural terrain, but to appreciate the necessity to improve the general musculature above that required to live naturally, in order to enable a horse to carry a rider.

The above points are explained more fully below.

(a) The first necessity for the foal is to understand to respond to commands from its dam. Like small children, foals will push behaviour to the limit, unfortunately human nature tends to regard this as amusing. Be realistic – it is not! Safety is of paramount importance, both the safety of the handler and of the foal. Taught early to respond as requested it will behave well and punishment will be avoided should the animal pass from one owner to another.

A badly behaved horse requires patience and retraining in how to interact with other species. This should not be dominance by the handler in the way described in the training manuals of the eighteenth and nineteenth centuries, nor should it be through subservient behaviour from the animal. Rather, the appreciation that there are certain 'rules' needs to be both understood and respected by both parties.

(b) Space, turn out, varied herbage, fresh water.

Horses living out enjoy a better life, and are in general healthier than those stabled. Cold is not a problem, as horses can insulate against cold provided they are dry. Modern turn-out rugs are very well designed to keep out the wet. Shortage of land makes continual turn-out living very difficult for some owners; wet ground becomes poached in winter and the tendency to divide paddocks into small areas reduces the natural wandering requirements of the horse which are associated with good digestion. Standing still continually when turned out is not what is required. It is interesting to note that research suggests the tendency for gastric ulceration of the stomach is less in horses kept out which are able to graze and wander, than in stabled animals. Research on gastric ulceration is still in its early stages but will undoubtedly lead to nutritional advice in the near future.

With excellent, responsible firms currently marketing herbs, variation of palatable nutrients is available; always remember, however, that if living naturally, the horse is seasonal in nutritional requirement. Could it be a mistake to ignore the seasonal pattern of requirement?

In the absence of a stream (see Fig. 5.1, page 41) or a pond, a constant supply of water is best provided by a field tank; buckets get knocked over, although standing the water buckets in the centre of an old car tyre reduces this problem. For those who feel drinking from a pond is dirty/harmful, it is important to remember that water may contain necessary minerals. Never forget the instinct to forage successfully is still highly tuned in the horse.

(c) A sheep or donkey to provide companionship is preferable to the horse being alone. Friends, in adjacent paddocks, are better than total isolation, although kicking out at fences in a confined area can be dangerous. The horse is a herd species and although when first turned out with other horses there will undoubtedly be a period of adjustment, the dominant group member will rapidly establish the pecking order. The removal of the hind shoes in group situations is advisable. Going barefoot is not an unreasonable idea.

(d) There can be no set time required to achieve perfect interaction with a horse. To have predetermined the amount of time required to train or retrain or to limit or curtail time is impossible. The amount of time cannot be specified, each horse is an individual. Just because horse X only took X weeks does not necessarily mean horse Y will follow the same pattern. This should be considered to be one of the most intriguing features of horse handling rather than as a nuisance factor.

(e) An understanding of conformation helps to avoid disappointment. The set of head and neck vary in every horse – some have long backs, some short and are described as being 'close coupled'. Books on conformation describe a straight or laid back shoulder, a trailing hind leg, being back at the knee. To understand conformation terms return to anatomy.

Take the scapula or shoulder blade as an example. The bone has a ridge or spine sited centrally that is easily felt. If the angle of the spine is nearly vertical, the horse is said to have a straight shoulder. With this conformation, the bones of the shoulder joint impinge one on the other early as the limb advances, constraining movement in the shoulder joint and so reducing the available length of stride. The horse with a laid back shoulder, where the spine lies at a slight angle to the ground rather than vertical, will be able to achieve a longer stride, the open angle in the shoulder joint allowing a greater range of movement within the joint (see Fig. 15.2). Early training should allow the horse to achieve a comfortable (for the horse) outline or self-carriage. Once this has been established, adjustments can be implemented if required or are possible always taking conformation into account.

(f) Left and right sides should be built as evenly as is possible and this is only achieved by working in straight lines. There is obviously a tendency to have a training goal; in many cases competition, and it is a common tendency to think 'surely it does not hurt to just try X movement at this stage'. However, endless practice of movements required in tests should be avoided until self-carriage, balance and the ability/fitness of muscles to achieve the movements, have been established.

(g) Horses do not canter, trot or even walk in circles in a field; they may swerve, performing a serpentine, but they do not circle. Working a horse on a single rein, even using two reins and asking the animal to circle requires the establishment of reflex responses to achieve unimaginable levels of balance and co-ordination. Too many unfortunate horses are incorrectly spun in circles before adequate development of

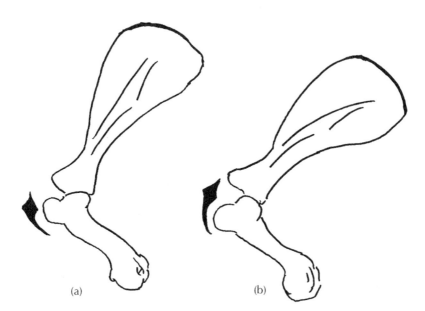

(a)   (b)

Fig. 15.2 Diagrammatic representation of the lateral aspect of a left scapula and humerus to illustrate the increase in joint angle between (a) straight shoulder, identified by a nearly vertical scapula spine and (b) laid back shoulder, identified by the scapula spine angled well off the vertical.

the appropriate musculature has been ensured. *Young ballet students spend years of muscle building to prepare their bodies before going on point.*

(h) Even if attempting to employ a natural approach to horse care, few people have access for exercising their horse in a situation comparable to that which can only be described as a natural gym, with facilities supplied free, courtesy of 'wild country', for example the prairie lands of North America, or desert areas of the Gulf and Arabia. The latter are not flat; dunes of sand, slopes, changes in footing, varied resistance secondary to the depth of sand, are ever present. Similarly horses bred as feral, and in early life left to their own devices, for example living on Irish bog land, in the Cumbrian Hills, the Welsh Mountains, the Alps, the Camargue, on Exmoor, are living in a 'natural gym' (see Fig. 1.1, page 3). When these animals are caught to be tamed/broken in, they have already built a strong frame, when compared to their domestically raised parallel, possess well-developed muscles and have achieved natural balance. They have no need to undertake what might be described as kindergarten activities. Once accustomed to being handled they are ready for first grade activities.

The natural gym

The natural gym provides:

- A pollution-free environment, both in the air or the ground. If these areas are present then horses will avoid such areas.
- Nutrition:
  - sparsity of vegetation;
  - choice of vegetation;
  - the ability to move from over-grazed areas;
  - natural water sources;
  - mineral outcrops;
  - exposure to natural sunlight.
- Muscle and skeletal preparation:
  - constant, slow movement to forage achieves motility of intestines for maximal nutrient absorption;
  - hills, inclines, soft going, deep going, hard going – varied resistance results in general increased muscle capability.
- Balance, secondary to proprioception stimulated by:
  - wide variety of terrain;
  - wide variety of footing;
  - the centre of mass is never fixed on uneven surfaces, every stride requires readjustment of balance. Balance is an essential requirement for survival, the equine brain is programmed to ensure the horse remains well balanced in the upright position. Varied terrain continually changes the centre of gravity necessitating balance adjustment in harmony with muscle activity and results in muscle building.
- Other physical benefits of the natural gym:
  - when moving loose, without tack and without rider weight, the horse has an unencumbered, freely moving back;
  - the position of the neck makes uses of the nuchal and supraspinous ligaments to maintain stability of the vertebral column;
  - the head in its usual position with the nose slightly forward, allows free passage of air;
  - there is no restriction of natural head movement, unlike most training regimes when the head is subjected to positioning by side reins.

- The natural gym also provides:
  - experimentation in company, developmental play;
  - herd behavioural requirements learnt, including submission;
  - abrasive areas to naturally pare feet;
  - space, providing the ability to slow down in a controlled manner rather than skidding to a stop if the horse is moving at speed;
  - trees or rock overhangs for shelter or shade (education of spatial awareness).

Natural muscle preparation

Text in italics suggests, where pertinent, either the horse's inherited methods of muscle use, or man-induced changes which curtail and/or ignore nature's building programme.

The horse is programmed to build without rider weight and all early work in the young horse, even when retraining the older horse, is best done from the ground. The basic tack worn by the horse is a snaffle bridle, a cavesson, a roller, and elastic side reins. The long reins themselves should be approximately 6 metres long. Their weight is important, too many long reins are too light. The use of long reins is admirably described by Sylvia Stanier in her books *The Art of Long Reining* and *The Art of Lungeing* (1993).

When training the horse, even when adopting a natural approach, it must be appreciated that muscle tissue requires preparation to achieve anticipated goals.

It may be useful at this point to provide a short reminder of the characteristics of muscle.

- The body is economic in how it develops and only prepares sufficient motor units within a muscle to cope with the demands of the current levels of activity.
- Increased requirement necessitates the recruitment and preparation of dormant muscle units.
- In order to build or condition, muscles must be exposed to increased levels of demand over a period of time.

It is difficult to achieve a multi-dimensional picture when describing complex muscle tissue. Muscle is not flat, nor is it a single tissue. Within its composition lie nerves, blood vessels, lymphatic vessels, along with many varied cell types. All these components are involved as muscles function. It follows that all these components will be involved and will be required to adapt as muscle is subjected to increased demands.

Each muscle is enclosed in an envelope, or sheath. Not only must this stretch to accommodate the increase in muscle bulk, secondary to enlargement as the muscle builds, but as the tissue interconnects with that of adjacent muscles, the result of targeting one area achieves multiple effects, and as no muscle ever acts in isolation, activity comprises 'group action'.

Muscles respond to loading relatively quickly provided the required nutrients are present in the diet, but remember the skeleton takes approximately 25% longer than muscle to remodel and adapt to increased stress or loading.

All muscle activity is under neural (nerve) control. Electrical impulses travel from the brain down the spinal cord. The vertebral column encloses and protects the spinal cord at every junction between the individual bones forming the column, a pair of nerves is formed, these pass, one to the right the other to the left, out into the body mass, there seeking and meeting other nerves. Then by joining together, they form larger, more efficient branches which eventually sub-divide into multiple, thread-like tendrils connecting to muscles. The sub-dividing occurs in a manner which enables agonist and antagonist muscle groups to receive messages from the same main nerve, ensuring instant communication to both groups.

The selection of active motor units within an individual muscle occurs in an orderly fashion and rarely is an entire muscle used. On demand, the number of motor units necessary to perform the task are activated. As they become fatigued, other groups within the muscle replace them in an imperceptible manner, allowing the fatiguing units to cleanse and refuel.

Conditioning muscle

If an animal is 'well covered' it is necessary to decide if this is because it is fat, or if its shape is due to muscle development.

Muscle responds and builds according to the demands placed upon it, but the ability to accept and cope with greater demands can only be achieved if certain criteria are met, or indeed if the animal has inherited the necessary muscle characteristics. Thus an animal mainly endowed with fast twitch fibres and which has been conditioned to working at speed over short distances, cannot be expected to suddenly work efficiently over a longer distance, its muscles simply do not have the capacity for such a sudden switch of effort. Its muscles will need retraining to optimise ST fibres and to improve and recruit convertible FT II/FOG fibres (see page 132 for fibre types).

When selecting an exercise regime, the type of activity as well as the speed, need careful consideration. The work of Snow & Guy suggests:

- Speed and power require a high percentage of FT I and FT II fibres (FG and FOG).
- Endurance requires a high percentage of ST (SO) fibres.

The pure strains of horses are genetically endowed with specific, breed related, muscle characteristics. These characteristics tending, in most non-TB and native breeds, to be a predominance of slow twitch (ST) fibres, but with sufficient fast twitch (FT/FOG) for a burst of rapid flight if required. Cross-breeding has created difficulties – which of the muscle characteristics of the two or more breeds in its genes has the foal inherited?

Response/requirement in order to condition

Conditioning requires regular and increasing activity. It cannot be achieved in one short daily exercise.

- Muscle takes time to respond to a new training regime.
- To improve endurance, the local circulatory supply must be given time to expand.
- The necessary energy sources must be available for conversion.
- The liver (a glycogen store) must have time to accommodate increased demands and improve its storage capacity.
- Heart and respiratory ability need to be improved.

To improve their capability, muscles require to be active. Early work with a horse requires, if possible, numerous short periods of activity rather than extended single periods, as the tissues need short bursts of activity followed by a short time to relax and recover. The ideal pattern is work, relax, work, relax. If riding out, this can be achieved by giving the horse a chance for a general warm up by walking the first mile out and then asking for collection, or perhaps, if on a nice wide track, performing a series of shallow loops, then letting the horse relax before again asking for an activity which could be described as 'an exercise'.

The natural horse is continually on the move, slow wandering is interspersed with short periods of effort.

Once fit, a horse will only remain in that condition if exercise continues.

The ability to work a horse in long reins is probably the most useful, freely available asset to any rider or trainer, but work in long reins should not to be confused with lungeing.

Driven in long reins, the horse is unencumbered by rider weight; if soft, only recently broken in or in the process of being tamed, perhaps just up from grass, changing disciplines, following an injury lay off or recently purchased, early activity can be manipulated according to the situation.

The horse learns to go straight and experiences light contact.

Driving in long reins not only exercises muscles, but is also a method of extending early communication between handler and horse.

Work should mirror natural activities, slow work over varied terrain, at walk.

Walking

Why walk? The head nod at walk involves and therefore improves the functional ability not only of the muscles at the base of the neck, but, as these inter-relate by connecting into those of the back, the entire musculature involved in back support, and so builds/strengthens.

Work on a lunge involves circling and the use of side reins, curtailing natural head/neck movements.

Other important effects occurring at walk include:

- slow work does not over-stress the skeleton;
- the bones do experience varied stress created both by muscle activity and ground impaction. The skeleton responds by remodelling, as long as nutrition provides the required ingredients;
- the deep muscles are activated due to postural variations secondary to changes in terrain, so the axial frame is stabilised by improved musculature;
- at slow paces, limb activity requires minimal muscle fuel, the stay system and associated muscles use energy-efficient stretch and recoil, effectively becoming correctly programmed.

If work over varied terrain is not practical due to a lack of facilities, for example where there is no open country, it is better if possible to use a field rather than an arena. One of the controversial European trainers, Dr Gerhard Heuschmann, a German *Bereiter* (professional trainer and rider) who is attempting to restore the principles of the 'old way of training', states that early training should not take place only in an arena. Horses require to be exercised, particularly in early training, on a variety of surfaces and over varied terrain.

Variation does not occur on the flat surface in an arena, where, once the horse has learned to balance it actually does remarkably little work. Once a horse has learned how to work on a nice, level surface it requires exceptional skill on the part of the trainer to increase the workload of the muscles.

Building the natural horse

Things seem to have gone amiss in the twentieth and twenty-first centuries. Regrettably, horses are rushed in their training. Today, three-year-olds are expected to execute a performance level not expected of a six-year-old in the days when 'old methods' were used.

Another consideration is the fact that the concept of early preparation required to stabilise the skeleton and build the postural muscles is rarely addressed in any books on equine education, neither was it mentioned in writings by the great masters of equitation. The reason for what might now be considered an oversight, is probably that there was no need to discuss early preparation. There was no mechanical transport as we enjoy today, horses *walked from their breeding grounds* to the schools of equitation. Many covered considerable distances. For example, the horses of the Vienna School came from the Iberian peninsula (Spain). This meant when a horse began formal education, it was well prepared from a musculo-skeletal point of view, and ready to begin serious muscle work due to the way it had lived for the first few years of life.

The methods described by Xenophon in the fifth century BC, were adopted by trainers such as Antoine de Pluvinel (1552–1620) and de la Gueriniere (1688–1751), who laid the foundations of what became known as the Classical School. While the age of the horse is not stated in the various treatises of the time, today, the horses of the Spanish Riding School, who follow these traditions, do not begin formal training until aged four, having enjoyed their early years on the Alps, roaming the high mountain pastures. This is when their skeleton develops, they build the muscles of stability and develop natural balance, all well before formal training begins.

Resistance

Natural training suggests trying to recreate the conditions required to build muscle without the use of formal exercises. To improve muscle capability necessitates making the muscles work harder. This is achieved by incorporating resistance, perhaps better described as making the task more exacting, through loading.

The constant change in the centre of gravity in the horse when it moves over uneven surfaces is a very useful method of loading. There are, as already mentioned, plenty of naturally occurring resistance features on open ground, to these can be added water wading and, if available, use of a beach, including the sea.

When being exercised, muscle, loaded beyond its metabolic capability, recruits dormant motor units, present within its tissue matrix, for it appears that all muscle has many motor units in reserve. There have been suggestions that muscle strength or competence may also be increased in a manner which causes an increase in the number of muscle fibres, this increase caused by possible longitudinal fibre splitting. In laboratory animals, this fibre splitting has been observed when the muscle groups have been subjected to very heavy resistance over a period of time. However the findings have been difficult to replicate in the human and as laboratory animals bear little resemblance to the horse it would be unreasonable to presuppose that this is what occurs.

Increasing the competence of muscle puts extra demand upon all other structures, for example, tendon, ligament and bone. As the skeletal tissue becomes stronger and adapts to the increasing demands, adaptation also occurs within ligaments and at muscular–tendinous junctions, these being the areas where muscle tissue changes its texture type, the fibres become compacted, changing their structural form to become tendon tissue. These adaptations take time and it is these which are essential before excessive training.

Loading does not necessarily increase the size of a muscle and certainly does not do so in early training. It should be appreciated that when considering loading, to overbuild muscle may be detrimental. This is because the equine skeleton is less able, because of its evolutionary mechanisms and makeup, to withstand the tremendous forces created by over-strong muscle.

Slopes

The design of the horse is such that its centre of gravity is sited forward. With the centre of gravity in the optimum position, the weight of the abdominal contents is evenly distributed, and the structures supporting the multi-jointed back are well able to counteract both their weight and gravitational force.

When the angle of body to ground changes, for example on a slope, the centre of gravity slides back as the horse goes uphill, and forwards as it goes down hill. This requires increased muscle activity in the muscles of the hind quarter masses on the upward journey and of the fore hand on the downward journey (see Fig. 15.3).

(a)

(b)

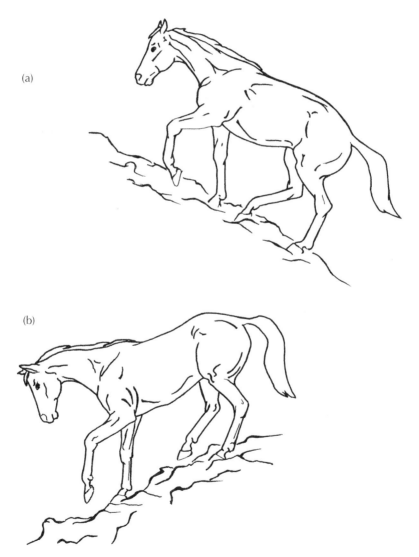

Fig. 15.3 Utilising the centre of gravity as a resistance. (a) Loading the hind quarters by going up hill – concentric muscle work. (b) Loading the fore hand by going down hill – eccentric muscle work.

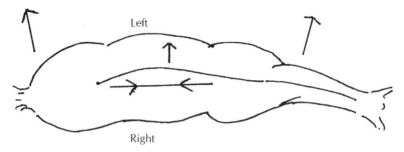

Fig. 15.4 Working the back muscles by going across a slope. Diagram showing the slight curve in the back secondary to the horse walking across a slope which falls away to its left. The centre of gravity has shifted laterally, creating the curve. The body is programmed to maintain a straight vertebral column, the muscles on the right side, are working to resist the force and trying to pull the column straight.

Muscles also work slightly differently during downhill work as they must lengthen or pay out as the limbs reach forward, rather than shortening. This type of activity, eccentric muscle work, is considerably more demanding than concentric work. If you want to know what your horse feels like after performing this type of work, run down a steep hill or walk down a mountain, your calves and thighs are working eccentrically. Register that unless you are super fit, the pain is not only that experienced at the time, but is also felt the following day.

The effort of movement, in response to the load sliding forward and thereby increasing the fore hand load downhill, and sliding backwards to load the hind quarter uphill, also helps to stabilise the frame, improving the stability of foundation upon which the working limbs rely.

On a slope, the muscles of neck and back are also subjected to loading as are their opposite groups, the abdominal muscles. It is not only limb muscles that build when slopes are used.

When the horse walks across a slope, the abdominal mass moves sideways, towards the downhill side of the body, creating a corresponding, slight lateral curve in the vertebral column. As the body is programmed to maintain the column as a straight line, the weight-induced curve requires increased work effort for the muscles on the opposite side. They contract actively to endeavour to straighten out the curve and maintain the correct vertebral alignment.

Working diagonally, back and forth, across a slope is a very effective method of improving the general musculature of the back (see Fig. 15.4). Interestingly, given a choice an animal chooses to work across a slope rather than go straight up or straight down. Look at any steep hillside and you can see the tracks made by animals, winding their way back and forth across the slope.

Undulating ground

This type of ground enhances balance perception. Each foot impact requires a balance adjustment by the horse, as the ground surface ripples, angles from side to side, and also goes up and down.

Balance is essential for safety. For those who follow the Three Day Event at Badminton, this type of going is found on parts of the cross country course and is almost

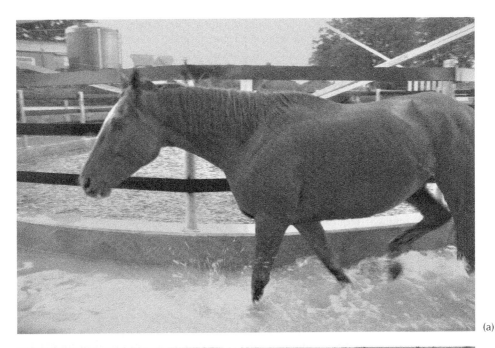

(a)

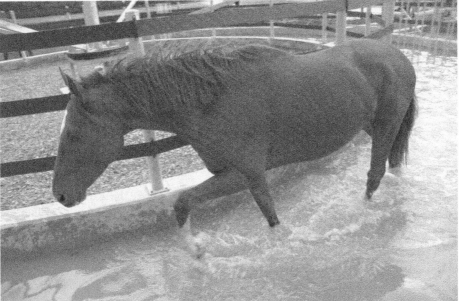

(b)

Fig. 15.5 The newly designed sea or water walker brings the benefits of wading to the yard. The water depth shown does not allow the normal overground limb swing, the horse must lift the legs. (a) The effort of the loin muscles is increased due to the need for pelvic stability to enable the leg lift behind. (b) The muscles at the base of neck are subjected to an increased workload as the head nod is accentuated to help balance as the front limb is lifted.

As the muscles of loins and neck are an integral part of the long back musculature the entire back support complex is worked hard as are the abdominals. Their activity is partly a reflex response, stimulated by the cold water splashing the highly sensitive abdominal tunic.

universally disliked by riders. However, the horses of endurance and long-distance riders, particularly those training on moor land, heath or the Salisbury plain for example, are accustomed to uneven ground and manage perfectly. Such ground need not cause damage if a horse has learned and logged the adjustments necessary. Damage occurs if the horse has no idea how to adjust. If adjustment were not possible most feral horses, particularly those roaming the vast tracts of Australia or the North American plains, would be crippled.

Deep going

As muscle adaptation occurs and the horse becomes generally stronger, riding slowly round the edge of a ploughed field (with permission) with the soil preferably harrowed to a reasonable tilth, provides excellent muscle loading. The horse cannot use the preferred, minimal requirement, of stretch and recoil. Moving the limbs requires short strides, lifting the limbs out of the dirt ensures work for the active muscles in their middle range, this is the recruiting/building range.

Beaches

Beaches need to be explored before being used, or at least walked over on a horse, before trotting, cantering or galloping, in order to avoid sudden deep patches or quick sands. Slow work in deep sand and/or riding sand dunes ensures excellent muscle loading. Many famous horses have been trained on beaches including Red Rum, multiple winner of the Grand National.

Sand not only provides a surface, which, with careful selection can be used for increasing the levels of resistance, but also, as the soles of the feet, the bulbs of the heels and the frog, contain balance sensors, these are automatically stimulated by the granular nature of sand.

Water

The newly designed Sea Walker (see Fig. 15.5 a&b) brings the ocean to the yard. The water depth is variable – fetlock-deep water levels create minimal resistance, mid-cannon deep creates considerably increased resistance. Both depths allow a muscle recruitment selection similar to that used for overground work, unlike the water treadmill.

Knee-deep water changes muscle recruitment from a limb swing to a limb lift. The muscles controlling the neck are recruited and the gluteal masses of the hind quarters work very hard. Due to the fact the gluteal mass sends forward a 'tongue' of muscle to the loins, wading knee deep is very useful if a horse is weak in the loin area.

Summary

The natural/wild horse develops slowly over a long time period, it also has access to varied nutrition, enabling selection of the correct plants at the appropriate time. Natural instincts enable the animal to seek appropriate minerals, and varied herbage for vitamins, when required. The body of the natural/wild horse is subjected to a wide variety of resistance but the animal is able to arrange the way it moves to its own advantage. Nothing in the way it lives is formal, prolonged or over demanding.

The domestic horse tends to be hurried – long distance, slow hacking and with few formal lessons, is a more natural approach.

Part IV

Exercise Analysis

16 The Classical Training Approach

There is a tendency, with reduced opportunities for open country riding, to have lessons. While many 'naturally' inclined riders may be reluctant to subject their horses to formal training and do not consider this is the route upon which they have embarked, if they begin activities variously described as flat work or schooling, they are using time-honoured methods not to subdue the horse, but to build it correctly as an athlete and so reduce the risk of injury.

Unlike in the human model, muscle activity linked to exercise with the purpose of improving equine bio-mechanics has remained largely unexplained. The first formal International meeting on Animal Locomotion was not held until 1991. Training texts tend to describe the result of an activity, not give the reasons for its use. The following example is taken from *Horse and Hound* (15/9/05) in the weekly, work-out series.

'Shallow loops-for straightening the canter.
In canter, many horses fall out through the shoulder while the hindquarters swing inwards. This exercise should straighten the horse, so it travels on two tracks and achieves self-carriage.'

No explanation is offered. Why does the horse fall out through the shoulder?

- Because the horse does not have the muscle strength in the appropriate groups to stop it falling out on a particular lead, even on either lead.

Why do the hind quarters swing inward?

- The hind quarters must swing inward to ensure the horse does not fall over, it adjusts its body mass to retain balance.

Why do the loops help?

- Because they target the inefficient muscle groups.

While every training problem cannot be due to inadequate muscle preparation a great number do stem from this. To counteract any problem concerning incorrect movement, riders and trainers would do well to first consider the problem from the anatomical perspective, and then select the appropriate exercise, either based on those of the Classical School or by selecting appropriate resistance activities in the natural gym.

If circumstances allow, it is comparatively easy to condition or build a horse for happy hacking even to pre-novice levels of competition in the natural gym. Conditioning, done without resorting to specialist exercises, results from careful selection of terrain within the working area, always incorporating graded resistance.

If circumstances do not allow, or if they curtail the use of a natural gym, the use of specialist exercises should be considered, particularly if competition is envisaged.

17 Surface Anatomy

You can learn to read the shape of the surface of your horse visually. This is known as surface anatomy. As muscles develop, their surface definition, particularly that of the superficial groups, becomes clear (see Fig. 17.1).

Stand your horse square. Standing behind him lift the tail, if you can see through between the adductor muscles of the hind legs to the teats or sheath you know your horse is weak in those muscles, you have read the state of the muscles by visualisation.

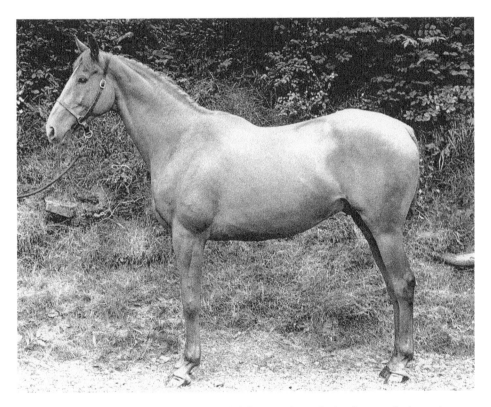

Fig. 17.1 The surface of the horse shows good definition of muscle development in the neck, shoulder, forearm, hind quarter mass, hamstrings, flank and second thigh. The back is also well muscled there is no appearance of a roach or tent shape.

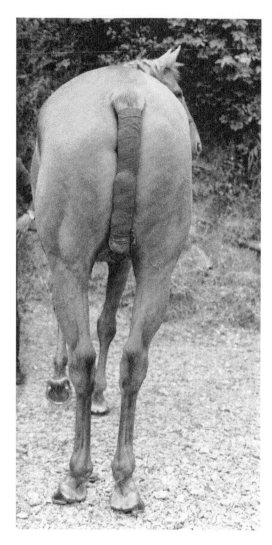

Fig. 17.2 The outline of the hind quarter muscle masses is uneven. The horse shows greater development in the muscle of the left hind when compared with those of the right. The adductor and second thigh muscles appear well developed in balance. This horse would give a good feel on the right diagonal, poor on the left and would have discomfort in the loins after exercise, secondary to thrust imbalance.

Perhaps the outline of the top of the hind quarter masses is uneven, one side appearing more or less developed than the opposite side (see Fig. 17.2). Decide which diagonal gives the best feel – left, involving right hind left front, or right, left hind right front? Exercises to improve the musculature of the weaker side require those groups to work harder. Choose an appropriate activity, then using it, position/work your horse for short periods to 'load' the weak muscles.

18 Specific Exercises

A good example of specific activities designed to target specific muscles and improve movement range, is the much discussed Rolkur. The positioning of head and neck employed in this exercise targets important, deep-sited muscles, involved in stabilising the junction of neck to body. The muscles pass forward from the ribs to join to the bones of the neck, bracing, amongst other areas, the front of the thoracic cage or chest. The front limbs, attached to this area, know when the muscles have developed appropriately, the limbs feel secure and are able to reach out, far in front of the body mass.

However, there is a big 'but'. Execution of difficult, specific exercises requiring precise positioning of body areas, particularly those involving 'rein' aids, for example the Chambon, is the job of an expert. Position the horse incorrectly and harm, rather than good may result (see Chapter 23, Artificial Training Aids Explained, pages 210–212).

Unfortunately, when building a horse a broad-fronted, common-sense approach is required. Choosing an appropriate exercise routine is rather like feeding, everyone has different ideas.

Factors involved in such an approach include the following.

Fuel – the supply depending on diet and general health

It is important to remember that the fuel demands of working muscle vary widely. Muscle activity at slower paces may demand more fuel than muscle working very fast for a short period. Activity also creates waste and this must be removed in the venous system. Those vessels depend upon muscle activity to assist in the transportation of their load.

The interchange of oxygen, essential for fuel conversion followed by waste collection, occurs as previously stated, in tiny vessels called capillaries. It has been calculated that between 4000 and 5000 capillaries are delivering to and removing waste *from each square millimetre of muscle* under athletic stress.

The commands to muscles are chemically induced via the ends of the controlling nerve, no muscle ever acts alone. All muscles work in a co-ordinated manner with the co-ordination masterminded by the intricate interaction of all segments of the nervous system. Training enhances the efficiency of neural ability. As the nerve enters a muscle, it moves into the tissue mass and forms the motor end-plate. This is a chemical command centre, it is chemistry which causes a muscle fibre to react in an active manner.

Chemicals released at the motor end-plate bind to chemicals already present within muscle tissue, the combination of the two chemical inter-reactions creates an electrical charge, which in turn triggers the chain reaction which allows the muscle tissue to convert its chemical energy into mechanical energy.

Improved performance therefore depends not just, as is often assumed, on working muscles to make them bigger and assuming that they are stronger, but also by creating an improved, efficient neuromuscular response through careful training.

Increased efficiency is also achieved by the fact that agonist and antagonist muscle groups receive commands from the same main nerves, this effects instant communication between them. It is for this reason that training must ensure that equal resistance is applied to groups that complement each other.

Why choose the Classical School?

The building of the musculature in the domesticated riding horse was well addressed by the schooling methods of the Classical Masters, whose use of a series of graded activities (exercises) spanning a time frame of several years achieved superb results, although it is possible the trainers of the time did not realise the reasons for success. Obviously, to follow their training programme in order and throughout, would not only enable horses to develop correctly but would also significantly reduce injuries.

The human parallel could be considered to be the dance student. The exercises of Classical Ballet prepare the body of the aspiring dancer, no matter their eventual choice of dance, through a series of graduated exercises performed as a daily routine over a period not of weeks or months but of years.

Considered anatomically, each exercise routine targets specific muscle groups, then, as stability, and correct execution of a movement, are achieved secondary to the improved functional ability of the targeted muscles, the horse or dancer progresses to the next, more exacting routine.

All movement involves the rearrangement of the joints of the skeleton. During movement, joints rely on support from muscles. If the muscle support is poor, or is in any way inadequately prepared, be it that of the axial frame, the appendicular levers, or both, joints restrict their movement range to that which they instinctively realise is safe. They only permit movement in the inner or closed range. As muscles develop their tensile capacity, in response to appropriate training, so movement range in the joints increases, the body feels secure, and the rider describes the horse as having become supple.

In today's world, if you wish to improve your muscular physique, you might choose to use a personal trainer, a person skilled in muscle development. If you wish to reach great heights with your horse, why not seek the services of an expert to teach you how to help your horse?

It is impossible to dissect each exercise used in the Classical repertoire to take a horse from safe basic movements to Grand Prix level, neither would it be pertinent for the content of this book. The exercises discussed here are the primary, basic activities, designed to stabilise the limbs, teach the horse to move forwards, backwards and sideways, safely and in balance, and then finally to execute a circle.

Common questions

When beginning work with an unbroken horse, perhaps discussing re-schooling, or beginning to try to improve performance, a number of questions spring to mind.

Q: *How do I know which exercise to use?*
A: Which movement does the horse find difficult? Watch the movement, mentally analyse the limb requirement. Ask yourself, is the frame stable? Are the all the muscles, including the stabilising and associated groups, adequately prepared? Is the footing at fault?

If the problem occurs when the horse is ridden, are you off balance, preventing the horse from feeling safe?

Q: *Which muscles are being used to perform the movement?*
A: Look in an anatomy book under the section describing the actions of muscle, this will help you decide the active muscles primarily involved. For example, horses which do not engage are not using their hip, hock and stifle to advantage. Attention to the hamstrings, and quadriceps is required, transitions down help.

Remember no muscle acts in isolation, group action is normal. Which other groups may be involved, perhaps the fixators. What range is required for the movement? Middle, inner, outer?

Q: *How do I know which muscles I want to get the horse to use?*
A: If possible watch the horse, have it work both to the right and left, analyse the problem. Is the horse leaning, using a shorter stride with one limb, swinging a limb out to the side, moving like a diamond? Which muscles are not doing their job? Then go to the anatomy books, work it out, choose the appropriate exercise.

Q: *For how long must the horse do the exercise?*
A: Unfortunately, every horse varies. Short, repeated sessions or sets are the most beneficial. For example, repeat an exercise a maximum of five times before a break, work in sets of five. This approach used at each exercise session over around a six-week period will usually suffice. Continue with an exercise for too long in a single session and muscle fatigue occurs; if you think this is nonsense try doing press ups for twenty minutes.

Q: *How soon will the muscles be strong enough to start to ensure the correct movement?*
A: Read the horse as you ride, they will tell you. Remember, they also have to instil the correct movement sequence in the brain, this will not happen until the muscles can execute the movement sequence easily.

Activity

Before starting any sort of training to improve muscle prowess it should be remembered *that gravity has provided a constant force, influencing the musculo-skeletal system from birth, and this influence was of sufficient importance for survival to ensure, even in an untrained subject, that the muscle competence of each animal will resist the forces of gravity exerted upon that individual.*

The greater the range of experience available in early pre-trained living, the better the muscle development when the horse begins formal activities. Resisting gravity ensured muscle development and this has achieved an adequately supported frame.

The pre-training period should, ideally, in the domestic horse, include handling. The animal should learn that interaction with man is not dangerous and should not be resisted and early obedience can be introduced.

Remember, because the horse is a prey animal it has a muscle co-ordination programme instilled for survival. Muscles automatically attempt correction the moment the optimum position of the body is lost or disturbed. This programme demands a straight vertebral column, the centre of gravity slightly forward and the thoracic cage suspended centrally between the front legs.

Changes in position affect the centre of gravity due to repositioning the abdominal mass. This huge weight provides loading (weight = resistance). It is these factors, the muscles attempting to restore equilibrium secondary to body reposition and with changes in the position of the abdominal mass, which provide the basis of selective recruitment for improvement of muscle.

Each gait requires different muscle co-ordination, each requires increased effort in the working muscle groups.

- *At walk* there are always three legs on the ground affording a good support base.
- *At trot* only a pair of legs is on the ground at any one time. The horse needs to co-ordinate diagonal activity in limb pairs; a two-base support requires extra effort and improved stability in the weight-bearing limbs.
- *At canter and gallop* there is a single support base.

An increase in loading is achieved by repeating each exercise at a different gait and also by variation in the pace of the gait.

- *Walk* on a loose rein, stretch, recoil, easy. Collection introduced, increased muscle effort.
- *Trot* horse allowed own speed, easy. Collection introduced, increased muscle effort.
- *Canter* horse allowed own speed, easy. Collection introduced, increased muscle effort.

Natural gym

Consider in the natural/feral animal that the distribution of weight constantly changes. Continual repositioning of the body, due to varied ground conditions, cause movement of the abdominal mass. A natural resistance is afforded by the body itself. As this weighty mass repositions, the postural muscles are constantly active, attempting to realign the frame and reposition the weight advantageously. This occurs in response to neural, brain initiated, commands. Each disadvantageous body position necessitates an ever-changing muscle recruitment, the muscles working against a self-induced weight.

This recruitment of muscle occurs continually as the horse moves. We know a wild horse would naturally cover up to a minimum of fifteen miles a day. The postural muscles are actively working, and thus conditioning, for varied time periods, the total work time depending on the time it takes for the horse to move fifteen miles – approximately four to five hours.

Working in the natural gym increase in muscle effort is varied by state of going and variations in ground levels. If the horse gets tired it rests.

Formal gym, arena

In the domestic animal, the postural muscles need to become active during movement but the arena has a perfect level footing so there is little or no redistribution of abdominal mass when the horse is moving straight. The body needs be made to change direction and create an abdominal shift. Working in the arena, variation is provided by changing body direction and later by the use of cavalletti.

- *A straight horse*: when preparing, and in order to avoid onesidedness, equal work for both left and right sides should be given.
- *The one sided, or crooked horse*: if the horse is one sided, or crooked, extra work for the less efficient groups is required.

While during early preparation in the Classical School, the horse is prepared without the inconvenience of carrying a rider. The exercises discussed here can be used either by working the horse in long reins, or with the horse being ridden.

The carrying of weight represents stage two in a training programme, ideally follow-ing preparation work in long reins. The postural muscles are always active but several groups must work either slightly differently, or with more effort, when resisting weight from above.

The postural muscles

All skeletal muscles are designed as identical pairs, one of the pair on the right side of the body the second on the left. Their function is to maintain the entire body in an optimum posture no matter the task required.

These groups that act as the nuts and bolts hold the bone frame together, providing a firm structure. They attach the limbs to the body and constitute the stay system.

The appendicular muscles

These groups form the stay system, attach the limbs to the body mass and move the body by converting the bones they control to levers. There are four directions of movement – forwards, backwards, and to the side, better described as moving laterally, both to left and right.

The brain programme of the horse does not expect the limbs to have to perform lateral work or circles; to swerve, yes, when the body is temporarily rearranged with the neck curved inward, the extreme side flexion is used for balance.

In order to achieve circles, exercises to target the ab- and adductor muscle groups are required. Read any Classical exponent, Podhajski, Klimke, Kyrklund, Heuschmann: once the horse has learned to go straight then lateral work begins. This activity changes the natural function of the ab- and adductor groups from that of acting in a stabilising capacity, a passive role, to becoming prime movers, acting in an agonistic, antagonistic capacity, an active role.

Back and neck

Longissimus: interconnecting individual muscles stretch from poll to dock, lying deep against the nuchal ligament fan in the neck, superficial from withers to pelvis, deep beneath the hindquarter mass. Involved in all movements of back and neck, they have a major supporting role to counteract rider weight.

Ileo psoas: in the loins, a group of muscles is sited within the body cavity, running on the under surface of the pelvis and lateral projections of the lumbar vertebrae. As well as flexing the sacroiliac joint they act as the major support for the loins and sacroiliac joints.

Abdominal muscles: there are *no muscles* on the under surface of the thoracic vertebrae, support of the area relies on architectural design, and nuchal ligament traction assisted by the abdominal muscles. The muscles play a small part in flexion of the hind quarter mass and therefore the postitioning of the hind limbs under the body mass.

The small muscles of the vertebral column (too numerous to mention individually) work in a stabilising rather than an active role; that is, they restrict rather than initiate movement.

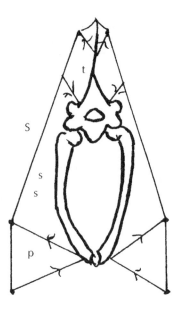

Fig. 18.1 The thoracic cage, forming the central section of the body mass, is hung between the front legs, s = scapula; t = trapezius muscle; ss = subscapularis muscle; p = pectoral muscle.

Early exercises

Straight lines, preferably without rider weight. The back musculature works as design intended. The head nod at walk is the natural way of involving the long back muscles. If riding, ride on the buckle end to allow head nod.

All exercises involve limb muscles; as collection is introduced, middle-range muscle work is influential in improving/conditioning the active muscle. Introduce collection slowly, the muscles will start to improve as they begin working in the middle range. Include stepping back during early work and ensure the horse learns to halt square.

The thoracic sling – trapezius, subscapularis, the pectoral groups
(see Fig. 18.1)

The thoracic cage is suspended from the withers by local muscles whose arrangement forms a sling. During body movement, the cage may swing up, down or sideways within the sling formed by muscle arrangement. The muscles act to restrain the movement of the cage. The sling muscles are also involved in adduction, functioning in partnership with the adductors, lying on the lateral aspect of the shoulder complex, as previously described. These groups work in partnership to ensure medial and lateral stability of the front limb both at rest and during movement (see Fig. 18.2).

The groups are of great importance during movement working, acting as stabilisers of the weight-bearing limb when it is advanced forward of the body mass and ensuring that the limb moves smoothly backwards in the same plane. (See Part III, Muscle Activity, pages 129–133.)

The ab- and adductor groups become, as previously explained, prime movers when their role is to take on responsibility for lateral movement.

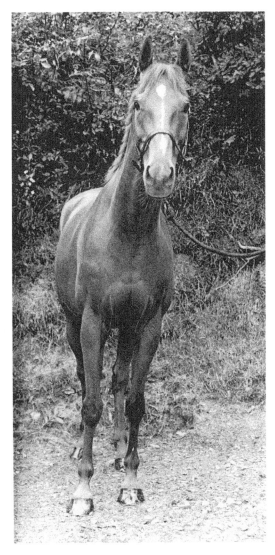

Fig. 18.2 The horse shows well-developed sling muscles. Visible are trapezius, the defined mass to the outer side of the withers, and the pectorals, sited between and on the inner aspect of the front legs, passing up to create the clearly visible masses on the lower chest.

Exercises

Once the horse has learned to go in straight lines, curves can be introduced, loops to begin with, then as the horse improves, the loops become sharper and serpentines are introduced (see Fig. 18.3). These movements marginally change the position of the abdominal load from central to lateral, the weight shifts first to one side then to the other depending on the slight body curve. The muscles of ab- and adduction, and all the muscles of the thoracic sling are also actively involved.

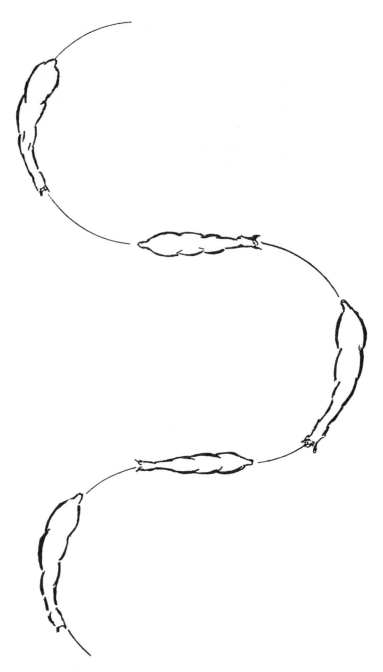

Fig. 18.3 Serpentines follow loops, they influence the ab- and adductor muscles of both front and hind limbs and encourage balance on a curve.

The gluteal muscles, the quadriceps, the hamstrings, tensor fascia lata, the adductors

The hind limbs attached via the hip joints to the pelvis are entirely dependent on muscle, for function and stability, other than within the joint.

The hind quarter mass is formed by the gluteal muscles, the outer flank by the quadriceps and tensor fascia lata. The hamstrings lie below the dock running down the back of the thigh, the adductors lie between the hind legs (see Fig. 18.4).

Just as in the front limb, the components of the stay system become active during movement assisted by the other muscles, each individual or group acting appropriately when recruited both to take the limb forward under the body mass, place the foot safely then initiate the thrust power required.

The ab- and adductor groups are influenced when performing serpentines, but become more involved during lateral work and, once the horse has learned to balance off a straight line, lateral work should be introduced. These muscles change their role, as in the front limbs, from that of stabilising to become the prime movers in lateral work.

Neither lateral work nor circling are a part of the natural horse's repertoire. While the ab- and adductor groups do develop in the natural horse, it is unlikely they would be sufficiently able, if developed in a natural training programme, to withstand the stresses placed on limbs when an animal is lunged on a circle. For this reason, the functional requirement of these groups should be considered and addressed by the use of appropriate activities if circles are required.

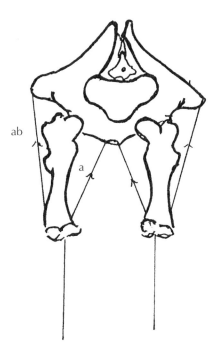

Fig. 18.4 The hind limbs attached to the pelvis via the hip joints are entirely dependent upon the complexity of the hind limb musculature for support. ab = abductor muscle groups; a = adductor groups. Balance between the groups is essential for maintaining the medial–lateral balance of the hind limbs.

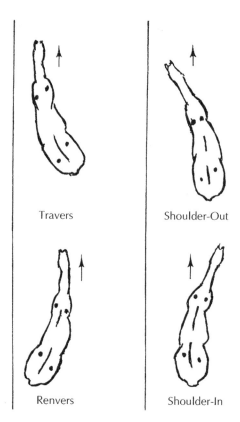

Travers   Shoulder-Out

Renvers   Shoulder-In

Fig. 18.5 Starting to prepare ab- and adductor muscles.

Taking the shoulders off the straight line can be used as a start, the side of the arena or hedge or fence all provide security for the horse in early stages (see Figs. 18.5 and 18.6).

Once the horse can execute lateral movements easily and correctly, the circle (see Fig. 18.7) and work on a lunge can be introduced. If the preparation for circling has seemed prolonged, remember the brain (computer) during lessons has to install a new programme. Every new activity must be imprinted. If the learning period is hurried, and incorrect programmes installed, the horse will react when ridden and asked to perform a movement learned in long reins, exactly as it performed when taught the activity in long reins.

Ridden work incorporating exercises, follows work from the ground, for success, the sequence of ground preparation should be adopted with collection added.

The description of the basic exercises should not leave the reader with the idea that these are the only form of activity the horse should undertake, they are a general addition to ridden work. The horse needs fun, time out from lessons, time to explore the environment with the rider. Formal lessons should only form a small part of ridden activities; when lessons are given, they should be included for short periods only to avoid boredom and fatigue.

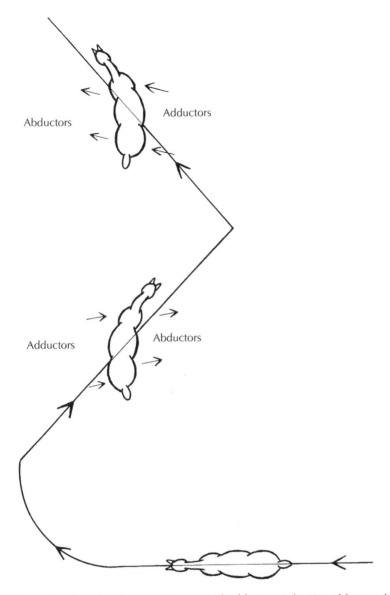

Fig. 18.6 Demanding lateral work necessitating considerable re-coordination of the muscles controlling the entire body.

Muscle problems, domestic living

Fatigue in muscles

Fatigue can be local or general:

- *Local fatigue*: a muscle suffering fatigue responds by reduction in capability. The onset of local fatigue may occur as one of a number factors:
  - a decrease in energy stores;
  - insufficient oxygen;

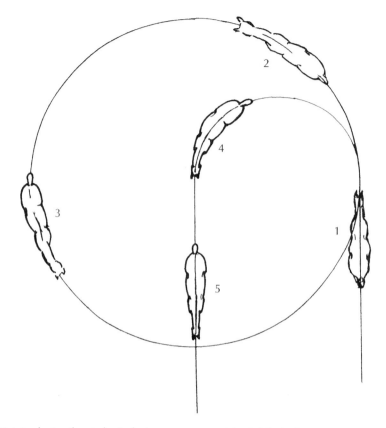

Fig. 18.7 Introducing the circle. 1: the horse moves straight; 2 & 3: the horse moves correctly, the track of the hind limbs following that of the fore limbs; 4: the horse comes off the circle; 5: the horse rebalances straight.

- a build of lactic acid;
- inhibitory commands from the nervous system;
- insufficient or inappropriate training.

Muscle fatigue is associated with local discomfort and a decline in contractile ability. Man is able to recognise and report the symptoms to his trainer, the horse will continue to try to perform as requested by its rider, recruiting other co-ordinations of muscle which are usually uneconomic. American research suggests that micro trauma may occur as many as ninety days before manifesting clinically. If a horse pulls out stiff repeatedly or suddenly is unable to work as before *look for a reason*. It is a great mistake to hope the problem will 'go away'. Massage or two or three sessions of exercises designed to target the area of discomfort will often solve the problem and prevent the establishment of inappropriate uneconomic movement patterns.

- *General (total body) fatigue*: this is the diminished response of the subject to perform to previous standards of even low-intensity exercise, despite being allowed a normal recovery period. The reasons for general fatigue require extensive investigation:
  - Is nutrition adequate?
  - Is there an allergy related to food?

- Are the haemoglobin levels within normal limits?
- Is there a problem with oxygen uptake?
- Is the body temperature reading above normal limits?
- Are the electrolyte requirements being addressed?
- Is the subject suffering from a systemic attack e.g.: a virus?
- Has the subject been overtrained/overworked beyond capacity?

- *Exercise-induced muscle soreness*: exercise-induced muscle soreness should not be confused with fatigue, the former occurring after unaccustomed activity or vigorous exertion. For example, training on good surfaces and in good conditions and then suddenly being confronted with deep mud, a strong head wind and high humidity.

  The associated discomfort and temporary stiffness will usually resolve within a few hours always provided adequate oxygen is restored to the tissues and circulatory flow stimulated. The problem can often be avoided provided a period of 'cool down' is incorporated into the immediate, post-activity period, for example, adopting the old adage 'walk the last mile home'.

  The complex metabolic processes associated with muscle activity give rise to many chemical changes and retention of the correct pH level is crucial. Chemical imbalance leads to a plethora of malfunctions.

- *Waste accumulation*: changes in metabolic processes can upset enzyme activity and eventually an incorrect chain reaction may totally suppress muscle contraction. Lactic acid is a by-product of activity. An excess of it may in some cases act as an irritant to muscle and cause stiffness and cramp. This type of cramp is not the cramp associated with 'Monday morning tying up' (see the section on Rhabdomyolysis, below).

  Excess lactic acid is removed from working muscle, as is other post-exercise debris, via the circulation. Normally, it takes between three to four hours for muscle to be cleansed, but light exercise following strenuous exercise has demonstrated an ability for muscle to convert the waste lactic acid into an energy substrate provided oxygen is present. Lactate levels in the blood are reduced more rapidly if the animal is trotted for a period immediately following strenuous work. Respiration and heart rates must return to normal before a period of trotting commences to ensure there is no oxygen debt.

- *Glycogen depletion*: the second reason for muscle fatigue is concerned with glycogen. Fatigue occurs rapidly when all the available glycogen has been used. Although fats can be used their rate of energy production is less efficient than glycogen and the muscles will slow their rate of contraction significantly. It takes approximately two days to replenish glycogen stores. Once again, light exercise has proved to be beneficial in the two days following strenuous activity for, just as with lactic acid removal, light work appears to hasten the process of replenishment. Massage enhances both lactic acid removal and glycogen replacement processes by influencing circulatory flow.

- *Rhabdomyolysis* (tying up): tying up is a complex situation and studies have elicited a variety of clinical profiles with variable findings. However, in all cases the muscle enzyme levels (CPK) are elevated, the gait is stilted, there is an acute pain response when affected muscle groups are palpated (most usually those over the loins), and the condition induces muscle damage. Unfortunately, once affected horses are likely to experience recurrent episodes.

  Although tying up was considered originally to occur as a result of the high lactate levels created by exercise, a Swedish study has shown affected areas to be alkaline rather than acid with the possibility that calcium might be a culprit. Calcium is necessary to control many of the metabolic activities during muscle contraction. As yet the pathophysiology of tying up has not been satisfactorily explained.

Summary

- In the early stages of conditioning it is both stupid and inadvisable to be in a hurry.
- Do not expect too much then every advancement will be a bonus.
- Think of the horse's brain as a computer, basic programmes are installed at birth, these do not include circling.
- A horse's inability to perform a new task can be due to muscle fatigue, or lack of muscle power or a combination of the two.
- All muscles perform better if warmed up before they work and massage is of great benefit in this situation. Post-activity muscle stiffness can also be reduced by massage.

Further reading

Back, W. *Development of Equine Locomotion from Foal to Adult*, Faculty Vet. Medicine, Utrecht University, Netherlands, 1994

Budras, K.D., Sack, S.O. & Rock, S. (Eds), *Anatomy of the Horse*, 2nd edn, Mosby Wolfe, London, 1994

Harris, S.E. *Horse Gaits, The Natural Mechanics of Balance and Movement*, Howell Bookhouse, Macmillan, London, 1993

Heuschmann, G. *Tug of War: Classical versus Modern Dressage*, J.A. Allen, London, 2007

Luard, L.D. *The Horse – Its Action and Anatomy*, Faber & Faber, 1956

Rooney, J.R. *The Mechanics of the Horse*, Robert E. Krieger, New York, 1980

Schoneich, K. & Rachen–Schoneich, G. *Correct Movement in Horses. Improving Straightness and Balance*, Kenilworth Press, UK, 2007

Skerritt, G.C. & McLelland, J. *The Functional Anatomy of the Limbs of Domestic Animals*, Wright, Bristol, 1984

Wynmalen, H. *The Horse in Action*, J.A. Allen, London, 1973

Part V

Overview of Training

19 Training Overview

When training, you are aiming to create a biological adaptation to improve the performance in tasks that are specific. Nobody becomes a competent or athletic equine trainer overnight but there has to be a starting point. This should perhaps be considered to be 'to aim to improve the physique and ability of each horse and each rider in order to achieve a harmonious interaction between rider and horse'.

Factors relating to fitness must aim to train the muscle to achieve the movement and then to train the movements to achieve the functional requirements. In order to achieve these aims it is necessary to address:

- strength;
- stamina;
- suppleness;
- skills;
- speed;
- specificity;
- mental attitude.

The complexities associated with muscle training were really not addressed until the 1990s. In 1992, Sahrmann stated that faulty movement could induce pathology, leading to trauma and also that musculoskeletal pain syndromes were seldom caused by isolated events but were the consequence of habitual imbalances within the movement system.

20 Faulty Movement

Incorrect movement patterns can arise from many things:

- habit;
- incorrect imprinting as described with the foal and the head collar;
- the inability of rider to command the horse correctly, resulting in imperceptible changes of function, incorrect movements in the horse, leading to imperceptible changes in rider balance also causing trauma to both;
- abnormal movements such as those achieved if the animal slips or the rider meets the horse wrong, in particular over a jump. Many people have stated that they felt their back 'go' as the horse landed;
- faulty posture caused as a result of sub-clinical pain;
- definite tissue breakdown or pathology.

One of the arts of both training the horse from the ground and training the horse when ridden, is to be able to identify and immediately correct any dysfunctional or incorrect movement pattern before it is logged in the movement centre of the brain as normal.

In order to achieve recognition of dysfunctional movements it is necessary to be able to rcognise and assess the inter-relationship between:

- the joints involved during the movement;
- the muscles required to achieve the movement;
- the nerve input.

This last point is because nerves not only command the muscles but also lay down patterns of movement in the cortex, particularly in the horse, which, as discussed earlier has a brain adapted to record movement patterns.

It is the re-establishment of the normal, economic movement pattern rather than allowing the continuation of traumatic movement which is one of the arts of training. This applies to both horse and rider. It also follows that early training must be specific in order to ensure that the movement patterns laid down in the brain of both horse and rider are those which are both correct and efficient. Response and adaptation in all systems will be secondary to, and as a result of, the training methods adopted.

Cardiopulmonary training

Consideration must be given to:

- training the heart and the lungs, the cardiopulmonary system, which is essential for increased stamina (IT training);
- training muscles in order to improve performance.

Improving muscle performance necessitates increasing both the time and the force against which the muscle must work. This is termed 'increasing the resistance or load-ing'. This cannot be achieved if the cardiopulmonary system is ignored.

As the horse progresses, it is also essential to improve cardiopulmonary function. Asking for exertion at speed burns glycogen rapidly putting the body into a state of oxy-gen depletion. Neural receptors are alerted and signals are generated, commanding the heart to beat faster to deliver the much-needed oxygen. At the same time, in order to ser-vice the blood requirement for oxygen, the rate of respiration also increases.

The heart is a muscle, and like all muscle tissue responds to progressive loading with increased efficiency. As the efficiency of the heart improves, it is able to pump out a greater volume of blood at each beat, the heart is then described as having improved its stroke (beat) volume. An increased volume of blood enhances oxygen collection and delivery, and the oxygen debt reduces. When the neural receptors signal all is well the heart rate slows, returning to normal.

Unfortunately, if the training stresses used to improve bone density, muscle activity and cardiopulmonary function are totally removed from the training schedule, after a remarkably short period of time, the competence achieved by the training methods begins to regress. It is therefore necessary to incorporate all the factors included in early training at least once every seven to ten days. This requirement is a relatively recent discovery and emphasises the need for a programme which to many must seem to include unnecessary retraining following a holiday or enforced lay off. Without an efficient heart (cardio) and without adequate oxygen (pulmonary) there is no hope of athletic competence.

Interval training

The use of short, medium to intense, bouts of activity, separated by short rest periods to allow partial recovery after the intense activity was used and proven as a conditioning technique for the cardiopulmonary systems of human athletes, by Roger Bannister in the 1950s. Refined and studied by successive human athletic trainers, the method is now know as Interval Training or IT. The short periods of intense activity create metabolic demand in the working muscles and to service requirement both heart and respiratory rates rise. The rest 'intervals' are designed to achieve a partial, rather than full resump-tion of normal heart and respiratory patterns. Before full recovery can occur, the next bout of activity begins, requiring as before, increased oxygen uptake and delivery to ser-vice muscle demand. While involving the cardiovascular and pulmonary systems, the method is also aimed at 'conditioning' muscle by stressing its metabolism and energy conversion. It is not designed to strengthen muscle, rather to increase muscle stamina enabling muscle to accommodate to the demands of increased activity.

It is often difficult to decide at which precise moment in an equine training programme to incorporate IT, for the limb structures must have been adequately prepared during the LSD (long, slow, distance) phase to withstand the requirements of IT. Each horse, like each human athlete, will require its own programme, the variables adjusted according to the final workload requirement.

Variables to consider:

- the distance covered between each rest period;
- the speed over ground;   A bout of activity
- the length of rest periods;
- the number of 'bouts' of activity/rest incorporated to create a set;
- the number of sets.

Some horses do not take to IT, fussing, refusing to settle in the rest periods. In such cases the Scandinavian approach known as Fartlek, roughly translated to mean 'play at speed', can be used. In this approach, horses are worked slowly over longer distances using the gait of their sport but activity is interspersed with short periods of high-speed effort. To many, Fartlek may seem to create unreasonable exercise demands, but using it is less troublesome if your horse dislikes IT. It also depends if you want a fit healthy horse rather than a partially fit unhealthy animal. Fartlek is nearer to the activities of the natural/feral horse – move slowly then a short burst of speed followed by a period of slow movement, and so on.

The Fartlek method is easier to incorporate into a general training programme, as IT requires a carefully calculated regime in order to be really effective.

21 General Considerations For The Rider

There is little point in implementing a routine to improve the athletic ability of your horse if you are in poor shape. Riding does not make a person athletic or 'fit', however, a fit rider not only rides better but is also less of a burden to their horse.

As with so many features in life today there are a serious number of misconceptions associated with exercise. People often have an unbalanced view of how to get fit, imagining the necessity for a health centre, even a home gym, with the need to spend time, often not readily available, pumping iron, fighting machines, until breathless, sweating and pink, not only in the face, but in the arms and legs also. *This is not necessary and not even useful.* Horses spend hours doing flat work, sweating and miserable. Far too many routines have been designed by people with insufficient knowledge of the requirements associated with physical activity.

The people who survive do things slowly. A survey of aspiring astronauts showed those who cycled to work each day demonstrated a higher level of general fitness when tested, than those who pumped iron in a gym. A similar result was observed in a group of NH jockeys, and regular golfers perform better at testing than intermittent gym enthusiasts.

A relatively recent report regarding a community in the New Forest, UK, hit the press. The local GP had persuaded people to walk or to cycle to the shop, to leave their cars at home unless going on very long journeys. The local health record improved to such a degree that health professionals are trying to persuade the public that regular controlled exercise is the answer to health.

If a gym is your aim then choose a programme involving circuit training. The late James Hunt was instrumental in providing a set of gymnastic apparatus, the Nautilus equipment, which required equal effort, both on pushing and pulling, during activity.

In order to ride, certain areas of the rider's body require consideration and the starting point before rushing off to classes needs to be a series of questions.

- What do you, the individual, wish to achieve both for yourself and your horse?
- Which areas of your body are important to target in order to improve/maintain present riding standards for yourself and to help your horse?
- Does one need strength to ride?

Homo sapiens developed as a hunter–gatherer with no conceived tasks other than survival. Species evolution is not in tune with twenty-first century living demands. The programmed facilities of natural man were geared to daily activity, moving over rough terrain to achieve balance, suppleness and stamina/endurance, these being the primary requirements for survival; how fortunate we are that we are all endowed with these primitive skills, of which few of us avail ourselves.

To ride you need to be able:

● to balance;
● to be supple;
● you require (just like your horse) muscle stamina *not* strength.

There is a difference between the long distance runner, who develops stamina, and the weight-lifter, who develops strength. Supple, pliable muscles are far more use to both rider and horse than strong bulky muscles. Stamina is required for the ability to perform repetitive movements over prolonged periods of time with only small changes of position. This is exactly what occurs in all riding disciplines, with the possible exceptions of show jumping and flat racing. In both of these disciplines, the competition time is comparatively short when compared to an endurance event, but both still necessitate balance and stamina.

Balance requires mobility, planning a riding programme, just as planning for any other sport necessitates that the exercises and stretches incorporated should mimic the desired function of the appropriate body areas. Mobility in the hips and stability of the low back are two key rider requirements.

Riding, unlike nearly every other sport, demands that both sides of the body work in unison. Training muscle co-ordination, joint movement and balance requires motor learning and neural adaptations to become equally bilateral. Many standard exercises performed in the gym are inappropriate, as they work first one side of the body, then the other, step exercises for example. Pilates improves body perception, but do the positions adopted mirror that of riding?

Joints needs early consideration due to the important communications which come from them which are essential to muscle activity. In man it is impossible to have a mobile ankle if the foot is stiff. Similarly, stiff ankles lead to stiff knees and so on, joint by joint up the body. Stiff joints also create problems by changing the manner in which the shock waves generated by impact are distributed and absorbed. Stiff joints do not allow a rider to be supple, balance is also compromised.

There is no need to spend hours of specially allocated time in a gym exercising and stretching, it is perfectly possible, and far more desirable, to build the necessary exercise activities into daily life. Long reining the horse goes a long way to improving riding ability, not by standing centrally in the arena with the horse going round you, but by driving the horse and working out of the arena, even if just in a field.

Riding requires bilateral work, if you always work throwing left when mucking out, do two left throws, followed by two right. It will be hard because one way is your chosen 'easy' way, but should make you appreciate it can be equally hard for the horse to work one side if the opposite is preferred.

Consider the implications of stiffness in the rider. Stiff fingers equal stiff wrists, elbows, shoulders, leading to tension to the horse's mouth. This stiffness may not be due to lack of muscle capability but may be caused by impaired proprioceptive function. Proprioceptors are neural messengers associated with the autonomic nervous system. Apprehension on the part of the subject can result in stiffness.

Reduced range in the hip joint prevents the rider 'opening their hips'. This changes the lower leg position leading to incorrect delivery of aids.

Walking over uneven ground improves balance perception; the arm position, when holding the lines (reins) should mirror the riding hand/arm position, relaxed shoulders slightly bent elbows, relaxed wrists, minimal contact for control.

Improving rider muscle

In order to improve muscle capability it is necessary, just as with the horse, to increase the workload. This can be achieved in a number of ways. Resistance is considered to be present when any dynamic or static muscle contraction is opposed by an outside or applied force.

This force can be generated during everyday activities:

- mechanically: a bicycle, static or otherwise, also good for balance;
- by positioning the body in order to lengthen a working lever (limb), running down hill, pushing the muck barrow, shovelling if you go both ways;
- using the subject's own body weight against gravity, walking rather than driving, not using lifts; walking up and down stairs as an exercise.

Part VI

Progressive Muscle Loading

22 Gymnastic Apparatus

Once preparation of the skeleton and stability have been achieved by the use of long slow distance, it becomes necessary to incorporate activities designed to increase the muscle work load in order to continue to improve the capabilities of the muscular system. To achieve this you will need to include a factor known as *resistance*.

Resistance is achieved by progressively loading muscle, by designing activities which require increased effort. The aims are to improve:

- muscle fibre recruitment;
- endurance capability;
- power;
- metabolism;
- capillary density;
- neural response.

To increase resistance 'or load' it is necessary to plan a programme and to incorporate a variety of activities which create a series of different tasks. In human athletic terms this is known as creating a 'circuit'. Just like the human athlete the horse should *not* be asked to repeat an exercise again and again and again, variety is *essential*. Could you go into a gym and do press ups for an hour?

Equine apparatus

The 'apparatus' for the equine gym is poles, cavalletti and jumps. Programme design, to create loading, is achieved through informed choice from the options available. Those available in the arena/school are:

- Classical exercises – long reins.
- Classical exercises – ridden.
- Ground poles – long reins – walk, trot, canter.
- Raised poles – long reins – walk, trot, canter.
- Small fences – long reins – trot, canter.
- Ground poles – ridden – walk, trot, canter.
- Raised poles – ridden – walk, trot, canter.
- Small fences – ridden – trot, canter.
- Grids (six or more cavalletti) – loose schooled, trot, canter.
- Grids – ridden – trot, canter.
- Incorporate changes of pace – transitions up and down.
- Changes of direction – circles, serpentines.

Progressive loading is achieved on open terrain from the following options:

- Grass slopes – lunge – walk, trot, canter.
- Grass slopes – ridden – walk, trot, canter.
- Road hills or grass – led off a second horse at walk.
- Road hills or grass – ridden at walk, working trot.
- Fences small – on the flat (ridden).
- Combination fences – small on the flat (ridden).
- Larger fences – loose schooled if possible.
- Larger fences – ridden trot and canter.
- Fences on slopes – ridden – trot and canter up and down hill.

In all programmes incorporate changes of speed, also relaxation/rest periods. A horse finds it difficult to maintain a shape for lengthy periods in early training, longing to stretch, relax, before trying once again to respond to requirement. A slow progression, choosing from the options available ensures obedience, balance and muscle adaptation.

Facts relating to exercise

Circuit training incorporates controlled activity, thereby ensuring 'adaptive changes' in muscle. Muscle, if forced to work in a manner necessitating repetition at low intensity, demands oxygen to enable it to continue its necessary aerobic activity. The result after a period of time is an increase in the density of the capillaries supplying the muscle fibres. Known as *improved vascularisation*, this increase in capillary density ensures both adequate delivery and sufficient amounts of oxygen can be made available should the need arise. If the long, slow activity work is not included in the early training programme, eventual requirements for oxygen essential for strenuous activity cannot be met and neither can waste be removed. This situation leads to oxygen debt and an excessive build up of both carbon dioxide and lactates, these may cause muscle damage leading to tissue *breakdown*.

Reasons for the inclusion of a 'circuit'

When planning any training programme the activities/exercises, both in the arena and on open terrain, need to be selected carefully to try to replicate the eventual functional demands the horse will encounter, and/or to improve the scope and capability of an animal already reasonably prepared but required to compete at a more advanced level.

It is impossible to write an exact recipe, each horse is an individual, each will respond differently, both in the time required to learn and for muscles to condition.

The circuit can be used to achieve:

- muscle endurance;
- muscle strength;
- body balance;
- obedience.

Endurance

To develop endurance following improved vascularisation, the active exercises need to be repeated over a prolonged period of time and against a moderate load. Steady hill work achieves this. As previously stated, muscle responds and builds to the loading it experiences. To increase loading walk straight up and straight down a hill, also work diagonally across a hill, working the muscles of balance, of the back and of the hind quarters, and when coming down hill, of the fore limbs. The activity experienced by the fore limbs when going uphill is not as effective at building muscle as that experienced when they work downhill. The work that the fore limbs experience as the animal goes downhill is eccentric work. As discussed earlier, this is one of the most exhausting and therefore the most stressful methods of loading muscle tissue.

Strength

Strength refers to the 'force' of output generated in working muscle. Strength training requires muscle to work against a heavy load for a relatively low number of repetitions. In the horse using the animal's body weight is the only method of increasing loading. Work jumping down a grid of raised poles at all three paces, walk, trot and canter, creates the effort required to improve muscle strength and therefore the force of contractile ability. Using a weight cloth adds to the weight of body mass, thus increasing load.

Balance

Maintaining balance while in tack is a lesson. We have already seen that the horse can co-ordinate within a few hours of birth. To balance after an hour or two of birth is not a problem; should the foal miscalculate, it is free to recover unencumbered by any form of restraint. Problems for the horse begin as soon as breaking-in commences, not just when the animal has to learn to carry man.

Tack is a restraint. It directs the manner in which the animal may move. Failure to move as the tack and manipulation of the tack by the trainer demand often results in pain, pain leads to tension, tension to anxiety. Each horse, just like each individual human, balances differently.

Working a horse from the ground and using side reins will begin to change the natural postural balance of the animal, a re-education necessitated by the alteration of head and neck to body mass. The rider will eventually communicate this requirement via reins and legs, as some flexion of neck is necessary in order to lift the back to carry rider weight. Remember that this stage is very difficult for the young or inexperienced animal. Try to put yourself in the same situation, envisage a situation where restraint has hampered your movement. For example, in a three-legged race, you are attached to another person whose movement and appreciation of movement is entirely different from your own, and only with skill and practice is it possible to co-ordinate.

The horse has first to learn to co-ordinate in a different body position, that is a position demanded by tack, and then to have rider weight added to its frame. No sooner has balance in tack been mastered than all skills have to be relearned, the addition of a rider requiring not only learning how to cope with an unstable weight, but also to co-ordinate new muscular activities. The groups adjacent to the multi-jointed backbone have to change function. Previously required to harmonise with and absorb tiny vibrations resulting from the forces generated as individual limbs met the ground and resist gravity under accustomed weight, the muscles must act to prevent the back from collapsing downward. At the same time they must assist in the maintenance of balance by counter-acting any instability created by rider weight moving laterally outside the animal's centre

of gravity. Obviously, if the rider is supple rather than stiff, skilful rather than apprehensive, secure rather than insecure, the horse will benefit.

You can experience what it might feel like to be a horse with a rider on board by playing 'horsey' with a small child, your back will soon tell you that it has had enough.

Horses raised on hills or mountain slopes have a better balance perception than those
whose only experience has been on flat land. Balance perception is essential, both for
performance and safety. Activities to train balance should be incorporated within general training; cavalletti arranged as a fan, slopes, direction changes, working on uneven
ground, jumping off angles all help.

An old-fashioned method was to secure a bag of sand to the saddle or roller while
working the animal from the ground, the horse learning to cope with the movements created by the weight before being ridden.

Obedience

Obedience is essential not only for performance but also for horse and rider/trainer/
groom safety and to avoid unnecessary injury. Obedience is not just compliance with
rider command, it involves all general behaviour. Just like small children, foals should
not be allowed to become domineering. They need to learn to accept restraint, to remain
calm when handled, led or tied.

Remember too that lessons should be short, for their attention span is similar to that
of a small child. Two- and three-year-old horses are like teenagers exhibiting a 'try and
see how far we dare go' attitude.

Early work in long reins is an excellent medium for discipline, acceptance of tack, the
square halt, not turning in to the handler when on a circle, stopping when told, backing
up, working over poles and cavalletti calmly, not rushing, refusing or ducking out.
Horses should not be allowed to snatch when offered a treat or a carrot, bang the door
when waiting to be fed, or bite the people working with them.

In the herd, bad behaviour is punished by the dominant mare, a swift reprimand soon
teaching the necessary lesson. Often a voice change from the handler accompanied by
one smart, light slap on the neck using the back of the hand achieves respect without fear
or resentment. Continual half reprimands, the use of whip or broom, do little other than
create irritation, fear or anger accompanied by loss of confidence and repeated incidents
of bad behaviour.

Some readers may consider these suggestions unkind, but the horse handled sensibly
will never be a threat. Allowing a horse to become assertive can lead to serious harm, not
only to those handling it but also to other horses. A boxer's punch is of Lilliputian proportions when compared with the striking forces generated by the limb of a horse,
neither does the boxer punch with steel knuckle dusters, probably the nearest equivalent
to the horse's shoe. They are classified as illegal weapons.

Problems associated with training overload

Overload describes a state when an exercise progression has exceeded the current state
of body adaptation. A useful method of detecting possible overload is through daily leg
observation and palpation (feel). Fetlock filling, knee filling, hock filling, extra warmth,
slightly spongy texture in place of a firm one, early minor splint formation or tenderness,
an early curb, all suggest programme loading has been too demanding or that insufficient

time has been allowed for the body to accommodate. Go back one or two stages, do not stop the animal completely, unless advised by your vet to do so.

Remember, it is better to vary, on a daily basis, all conditioning routines and thus minimise the risk of overload as a result of continuous repetition which may cause fatigue.

In the human athlete, scientists in the USSR demonstrated that the maximum number of repetitions for any single training activity in an exercise session should not exceed seven. Fatigue is complex and describes the diminished activity of muscle tissue to respond to an activity stimulus. This diminished response is a multi-factorial problem. Amongst the many factors involved, are a decrease in energy store and/or supply, a build-up of lactic acid, insufficient oxygen delivery, and an inadequate circulatory network.

Fatigue occurs if muscle has not been allowed time to accommodate to a particular exercise demand, especially if the increase in capillary bed did not occur, because the early programming designed to ensure the adaptive response of increased vascularity was either hurried or omitted. Damage to muscle occurring as a result of fatigue is a serious problem, motor units self-destruct and often recovery is by scarring, which reduces the capability of the affected muscle group for all time.

Recovery from exercise

Adequate periods of time to allow recovery following exhaustive exercise sessions should be built in to every training programme. Muscle requires time to replenish the energy utilised during exhaustive exercise, to rebuild tissue damaged during exhaustive exercise. Scientific studies show that light exercise, performed during the periods allowed for recovery, enhances the eventual recovery, thus the owner/rider should consider exercising the horse at an exhaustive level for three continuous days, followed by three to four days of light exercise to avoid excess demand. Studies, both from North America and Australia addressing equine recovery suggest that on the day following competition the horse should be walked slowly for approximately one hour, or put on a horse walker twice for two, half-hour periods. They should also be turned out for two to three hours, weather conditions permitting.

On day two, the horse should be exercised, at a brisk pace, for up to one hour, combined with being turned out, weather conditions permitting. It appears that day three is the critical day for recovery and this is the day on which the horse should be allowed total rest, this comprising no ridden activity but, weather permitting, turned out into a paddock before recommencing normal training on day four.

Many of the new studies have addressed endurance and as all concepts of muscle recovery have, until recently, been taken from that understood to occur in the human athlete, the increased interest in equine sports physiology will, as more studies are conducted, prove or disprove the human-based theories. Until this research is conducted, there can be no hard and fast rules concerning fatigue and recovery but an intuitive owner/rider will read their horse and should be able to assess the level of fatigue experienced and the level of recovery achieved.

Turn out to aid recovery

Turning a horse out to grass is not unkind, every horse should be allowed the freedom to move, roll, graze unrestricted. Unfortunately, many paddocks are over horsed, resulting in the destruction of pasture particularly in wet weather. People lucky enough to own grazing will find their horses are healthier and easier to keep and handle if the animals spend several hours a day out. Once the routine has been established, horses do not gallop madly around when freed.

New Zealand rugs are excellent for turn out, in cold or wet conditions the neck extension is essential. Field sheds are rarely used but are useful for haying in winter to avoid trampling.

The late Captain Tim Forster, the well-known National Hunt trainer, trained many of his stars from the field as do all the New Zealanders. It is normal procedure in New Zealand where all competition is just as demanding as in the Northern Hemisphere, and the climate not dissimilar, so why change?

It is amusing to note that, in 2000, when asked by BHS examiners what they did to their horses following International Three-Day Events, a trio of grooms, then world leader event grooms for the NZ Olympic Team, chorused, 'turn them out'. Apparently, they nearly failed their exams, their approach being considered negligent. This is *not so*, it is a more natural approach.

Gymnastic exercises using long reining, lungeing or work in hand

Long reins

All the great masters of equitation taught and still teach horses using long reins. There are four schools of long reining, each requires the use of two reins but the angulation of reins to operator is different in each school. The English method is probably the most practical unless the person working the horse has been trained by a Master of the Classical School.

Long reining is an excellent way for the trainer to enhance his or her own pre-season fitness campaign for the trainer must walk. The tack is identical to that used when lungeing, snaffle bridle, cavesson, roller, elastic side reins but two rather than a single line are required.

The horse is tacked up in snaffle bridle, elasticated side reins running from snaffle ring to the roller, on which three or four sets of rings are mounted at various heights from the girth attachments. A cavesson with three rings on the noseband serves as the anchor point for the reins. In the English method, the inner rein, attached to the inner cavesson ring, passes directly to the trainer's hand. The second, attached to the outer cavesson ring, continues on the far side of the horse; the outer rein is passed through a chosen ring on the far side of the roller. The rein continues until passing behind the hind quarters (under the tail) lying 20–30 cm (9–12 inches) above the hocks. The rein continues to the trainer who should have one rein in each hand. The horse is driven between the two reins, the trainer positioned slightly behind, to the inner side, of the hind quarters of the animal (see Fig. 22.1).

The reins should exert the same pressure as if the animal were being ridden. The inner rein controls direction, the outer assists in the balance of the hind quarters. Changes of direction can be incorporated although this necessitates adjustment of the inside rein which must be threaded through a ring on the inner side of the roller at a height similar to the outer rein. It takes a little more practice to work this way and a novice handler will require help from an expert.

The addition of lateral work will increase the gymnastics of any exercise programme in a manner difficult to achieve by a novice working a horse on a lunge. The introduction of cavalletti further increases gymnastic scope.

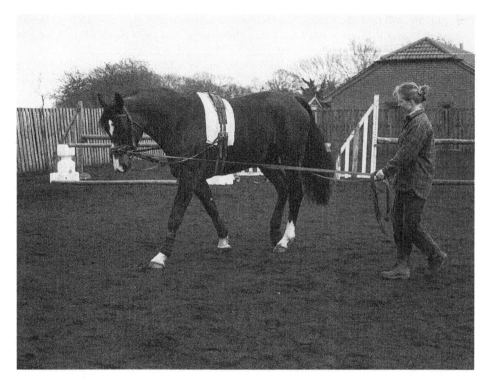

Fig. 22.1 A horse working in long reins. The trainer is walking with the horse positioned just behind the inside hind quarter. The side reins are not restricting the normal head nod, nor forcing an outline. The outside rein is controlling the hind quarters. The inside rein has a shade too much tension for perfection.

Effects of long reining

Long reining enables the muscles to build unencumbered by a rider, the back can work as nature intended. Long reining teaches balance, co-ordination, change of direction and encourages the horse to go forward.

Lungeing

Sadly, today's understanding of lungeing is to put on a bridle, with a single rein to the bit, and then teach the horse to circle around the trainer. This method is of little or no benefit to the horse as it spins like a whirling dervish on the end of the lunge line. This is not lungeing. Unfortunately, the 'dervish' spin tends to be not the exception but the rule, particularly when the trainer is trying to lunge in a large arena, in a paddock, or pre-competition, in an open area.

Lungeing is viable in a lungeing ring, where the outer perimeter of the circle, usually high sided and boarded in, enables the horse to be controlled within a circle of set parameters. The size of lungeing rings vary but the average lunge line is 6 m or 20 feet in length and the animal should be encouraged to work on a large circle. The imbalance achieved by an untutored or immature animal working on a small circle does more harm than good. Nearly all European lungeing methods employ both a handler and an assistant.

The activities concerned with lungeing are considered to be far more complicated than those concerned with long reining. When lungeing, the handler must keep the horse

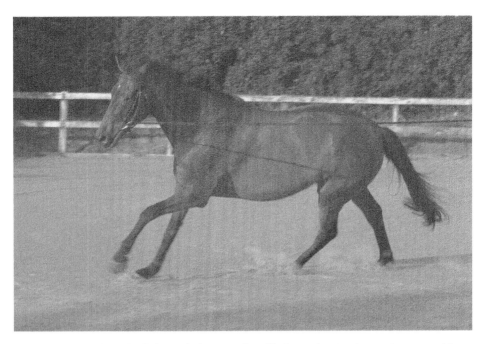

Fig. 22.2 A horse being badly lunged. The animal is off balance, leaning in, running not working. The trainer is probably 'fixed to the spot'.

between lunge line and whip, ensure no lateral head tilt occurs, ensure the hind limbs track in line with those of the forehand and ensure perfect balance and maintain cadence (see Figs. 22.2 and 22.3).

The tack used should be a cavesson, with or without side reins, with these attached if used, from bit to roller or saddle. The single line or rein fastened preferably to the central ring of the cavesson. If side reins are employed, care should be taken to make certain they are fitted in a manner that allows the natural outline of the horse to be retained until the animal has settled.

It should never be forgotten that in early training many experiences are new to the horse, no matter if the horse is being prepared from the ground or with a rider on its back. If a horse taught to trot or canter from the ground over bends, going behind the bit, why should it change its way of going when ridden at trot and canter? It is essential to achieve from the ground that which will be required when riding commences, reprogramming is very difficult.

The reason that many of the European masters of equitation, both past and present, have built horses from the ground is to ensure that the musculature is fully prepared and the activity learned before the animal is asked to carry rider weight. To work a horse from the ground correctly, when not in a 'lunge' ring, requires considerable practice. Far too many horses, even in a ring and correctly tacked up, are allowed to rush, 'motor biking'. They lean in, tracking incorrectly, the hind legs making their track away outside that of the fore legs. This is not working or learning, just teaching bad habits. Whenever working, as discussed in the previous paragraph and in the imprinting section, a horse learns to move in the way it either adopts for comfort, or is made to use. Retention of a movement co-ordination does not take long to become habitual, but it takes a long time to unlearn the habit and to establish a new set of movement parameters.

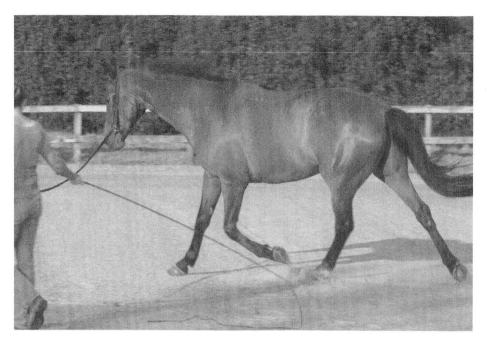

Fig. 22.3 A horse working correctly on a lunge. The horse is balanced between rein and whip, the trainer is moving with the horse.

'Tying' the horse into a shape when first on the lunge achieves nothing, as the animal learns to 'lean', using whatever device has been used, in order to balance itself. The situation is similar to that of a child who has learned to ride a two-wheel bike using stabilisers. Remove the stabilisers and the child will wobble and fall, balance must be relearnt addressing the new situation. Begin by letting the horse learn to balance without restraining aids, other than possibly a pair of loose side reins. Gradually introduce the restraint preferred to achieve the new position 'demanded'.

Most gadgets tend to create flexion only at the poll. This is not acceptable as the hind quarters merely 'tuck' and the animal trails the hind legs. Remember, there are two ends and a middle to consider! When watching horses who are working behind the bit with an exaggerated flexion at the poll, nose somewhere near the chest, active front limbs but showing little hock activity and with a hollow back, it is obvious that these animals have learned and logged an incorrect position. When working from the ground, be careful never to restrain to such a degree that forward movement is constrained. It is preferable, unless you are an expert, to work off the cavesson rather than the bit. A roller is prefer-able to a saddle and adjustable side reins, partly elasticised, should run from a snaffle bit to the roller.

It is difficult for a novice, whether the novice be the trainer or the horse, to achieve work using lungeing. Remember, exercise is not work. It is also very difficult, almost impossible, to achieve a perfectly balanced circle in an untutored animal if the trainer is not practised in the art of using a lunge. As in any work programme, begin at walk, progress to trot and finally to canter, when balance and evenness of pace have been achieved. Try to work the horse by voice command, in preference to flicking the lunge whip. The whip should be used for guiding *not* for painful encouragement or punishment.

Effects of lungeing

Correct work on the lunge builds the muscles of back and loins particularly the postural muscles closest to the back, named, as in the human, the multifidi. Although the equine back is designed to be loaded, the abdominal contents and gravity exert a downward force which the multi-jointed vertebral column must resist. When rider weight is added, the postural muscles need to increase their isotonic capabilities to avoid the back hollowing or ventro flexing.

In a riderless horse, these muscles act to ensure that the necessary rigidity of the main frame is sustained, for the back forms the central strut of the body mass. To enable the hind limb thrust to push the total body over the planted fore limb, back movement must be reduced to a minimum.

The lateral joints of the equine back also ensure stability, side bending is not catered for in the anatomical design. The mechanical angles present in the joints from base of neck to the junction of back to pelvis are not constructed in a shape which allows side bending, neither are there any muscles to achieve a pure side bend. In order to execute such a movement the entire mid section of the equine vertebral column must rotate. This movement is uneconomic for survival in the wild so the postural reflexes of the equine resist the rotational torque continuously, the local muscles working to retain the straight flexible rod. Circling creates this torque thereby activating the small anti-torque muscles. Over time this improves their tone, and thereby improves the ability of the horse to carry rider weight.

If the neck is left free on a lunge, the musculature works as nature intended. If the head is positioned by severe restraint, the neck musculature has to learn to work to hold the position. Static muscle work required is very demanding. Head and neck normally enjoy the elastic recoil of the nuchal ligament with muscle activity minimal for energy conservation. With the head restrained in an abnormal position, this normal elastic recoil is not available for maintenance of the cervical curve or to prevent the head being pulled downward by gravity. If the neck muscles are forced to support the weight of the head and also resist gravitational pull, the musculature must work in an isometric fashion, largely in the inner range. This is extremely tiring due to the muscle fatigue created. After a minimum of three to five minutes, restraint should be removed, the horse allowed to stretch its neck and to work enjoying the elastic recoil of the nuchal ligament, thus enabling the muscles to refuel and recover before the restraint is reapplied.

On a lunge, the limb muscles have to learn to balance the body weight over the limbs on the inner side of the circle and to adjust all limb movements to avoid limb collision. The muscles of the hind limb on the outer side of the circle deliver the greatest thrust, they are working concentrically and are required to achieve enough power, in middle range, to propel the body mass with little help from the inner hind quarter, these muscles working in their inner range mainly eccentrically.

To *work* correctly on a lunge is an excellent gymnastic activity, but no horse should continue this activity for longer than fifteen minutes at a time, it must be allowed recovery periods.

As the horse becomes proficient and balanced, the inclusion of a line of poles, later raising the poles and then converting them to cavalletti, introduces progressive loading. The distance between individual poles must be adjudged by the rider in conjunction with the length of stride of the individual animal. Of course, the distances must constantly be adjusted because there are different requirements at each pace.

Animals that have become used to voice command can be loose schooled, even incorporating poles. Jim Grant's 'Rosie', one-time member of the United States Three-Day Team, was a perfect example of this. Jim stood in the middle of an arena with poles arranged at various strategic points and directed Rosie by voice alone.

The mistakes made by those unskilled in lungeing are to:

- allow the horse to rush;
- allow the horse to lean in;
- allow the horse to work on two tracks;
- allow the horse to choose its own pace;
- imagine the horse is 'working' as it ambles or runs.

Work in hand

To work a horse in hand, the rider or trainer is positioned just behind the horse's head nearly level with its shoulder. One hand holds the reins just below the bit and the other, a long dressage whip. The whip is held in the manner of a fencing foil and employed, as described by Linda Tellington-Jones, in her treatise on wanding (1999). The method is a very valuable aid in training, the horse learning to collect himself, round the back, work in balance and most important engage from behind. Lateral work, square halts and rein backs are also achieved using this method.

Exercises in hand are performed in walk and at trot, the aim of the trainer working the horse being to achieve gentle restraint, by the use of the hand on the reins, at the same time encouraging forward movement by gentle tapping with the whip, either in the exact position where leg aids would be applied, or by touching the horse's thigh. The horse is usually wearing normal tack, its saddle and a snaffle bridle.

Work in hand is commonly used in Europe, but there are few trainers in the UK who employ the technique, although building, balancing and collecting before rider weight is added have enormous advantages. Done correctly over a period of time, the performance of horses worked in this manner will improve dramatically.

To summarise:

- long reining teaches balance, co-ordination, change of direction and encourages the horse to go forward;
- lungeing is used to teach limb co-ordination, to build back muscles by the use of the circle and to selectively load the outer limbs;
- work in hand achieves collection and forward impulsion;
- it is also possible to achieve, eventually, the brilliant muscle building afforded by piaff, but in the Classical world this starts in pillars.

The use of poles and cavalletti

Poles

Poles can be used to:

- vary stride length;
- improve joint proprioception;
- improve muscle co-ordination;
- re-establish balanced limb activity following injury.

Vary stride length (see Fig. 22.4)

Teach the horse to go over one pole at walk and trot before laying out a complicated grid or fan. Distances between poles are always an issue for debate as every horse has a different stride length and conformation will determine the length achieved. A horse

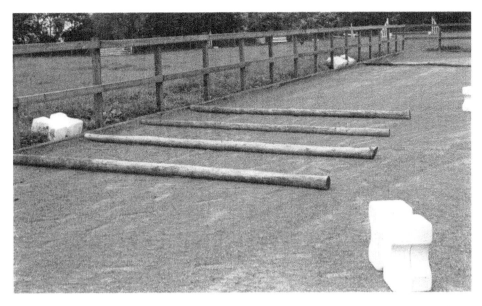

Fig. 22.4 Poles are used to achieve variation in stride length and so change the range of muscle activity.

with a good sloping shoulder will be capable of a far larger stride than that of a horse with a straight shoulder. To calculate a distance applicable for and fair to an animal, walk it down the long side of a freshly harrowed school and measure the distance between the imprints of fore and hind feet. Do the same at trot. Progress from one to two poles then up to four and finally to six. Change the distances between the poles to vary both length of stride and pace. The horse works harder at middle paces than at extended paces when the elastic recoil of ligaments aids activity.

Improve joint proprioception

Joints are loaded with sensors known as proprioceptors. These sensors communicate with the centres of movement co-ordination. The greater the variety of experiences the joints encounter, the wider the proprioceptive appreciation. Variation is provided by fans of poles and varied distances, either between poles in a line or between poles on opposite sides of the arena.

Improve muscle co-ordination

Canter down one side of the school, trot down the other, with poles arranged to be incorporated with the horse on a circle; every variation tests co-ordination as the individual limbs learn to move in a variety circumstances to avoid collision with either the poles or each other. The horse has four limbs to co-ordinate and the centres in the brain, from where movements initiate, are pre-programmed to avoid contact between a hind foot and fore leg. Severance of a tendon in the wild is catastrophic for survival.

Horses do on occasions over reach or clip a fore leg with a hind. Good co-ordination, achieved by keeping training varied helps to reduce the risk.

Re-establish balance limb activity

A horse which hurts, even if the pain is subclinical, will alter its movement patterns to avoid pain. A horse hurting in front will shorten its stride, a series of short strides reduces the weight bearing period on each limb. How often does one hear, 'he/she used to move like a dream, now look, no stride at all'. Once the reason for the change in stride has been sought, found and removed, the short stride will remain, it has become the 'accepted' movement for the horse. Work over poles, starting with them close together and gradually increasing the distance will, over a period of time, restore the original stride pattern through re-education. Pole work can be both from the ground and ridden.

Cavalletti

Cavalletti are poles raised off the ground 15–20 cm (6–8 inches). They are either purpose built or constructed by using two blocks, available from most horse requisite centres, and a pole.

Cavalletti work achieves:

- co-ordination – horse and rider;
- balance – horse and rider;
- muscle strengthening – horse and rider;
- discipline of movement – horse and rider;
- preparation for jumping fences – horse and rider.

The horse imparts a different feeling at each pace secondary to its balance requirements, four gait, two gait and these gait sequences all necessitate varied limb co-ordinations and balance variation. The rider must adjust to these variations in an imperceptible manner in order to avoid putting the horse off balance (see Fig. 22.5 a&b).

Muscle strengthening

Grids progressively load equine muscle as the horse works to lift its legs so that they clear the poles. The rider will begin to implement and fine tune the closed-chain reflexes discussed during rider preparation, when isometric activity for the lower limbs was considered. Rider rhythm is also involved when riding down a grid.

Cavalletti work should not be continued for more than a maximum of fifteen minutes. At the conclusion of concentrated lessons, the horse could be taken out for its normal long, slow hack.

As both rider and horse become more confident over the lines of poles, the distances should be adjusted in order to either lengthen or shorten stride, and small fences introduced at the end of a line of poles.

Discipline of movement

Work in an arena is contained work requiring a disciplined approach, partly necessitated by the space available but also because the activities are lessons not just work. Repetition, the spacing between the cavalletti and the number of cavalletti require control, concentration and effort to negotiate successfully.

Preparation for jumping fences

To jump fences successfully horse and rider must be in harmony. During the movement leading up to the fence, the rider may need to achieve restraint to meet it correctly but at no time should the rider interfere with the horse when it is in the air. To achieve this is a very big learning curve. Small fences can be constructed using cavalletti enabling the rider to extend their experience before progressing to greater heights and starting to school over fences.

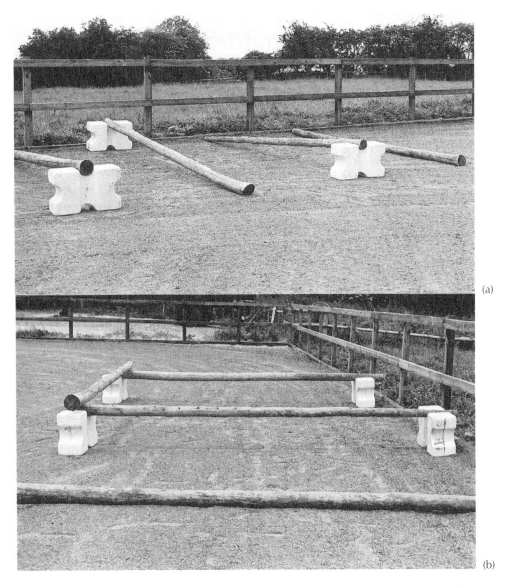

(a)

(b)

Fig. 22.5 a&b Variously arranged cavalletti. Arrangement should be varied in order to achieve the required outcome.

A pole placed across the gate so the foal or young horse must go over it when leaving the field, begins to imprint the balance requirements for eventual jumping. When eventually ridden away, use small logs in woodland to increase the imprint range, trot over the obstacles first, then eventually canter.

23 Artificial Training Aids Explained

Training Aids were designed/invented by past great masters of horsemanship. There is a great variety and all undoubtedly have a use. Unfortunately, however, they may be incorporated into training at a very early stage, usually before the horse has been worked sufficiently to build an adequate musculature to enable it to achieve the position enforced by the aid naturally. Many problems associated with position of head, neck and back are created rather than cured by the inappropriate use of an 'aid'.

The modern concept of an 'aid' seems to be that they are designed for changing the position of the horse's head and neck in an endeavour to put the horse into what is assumed to be a correct outline. Just as it is quite impossible to achieve an exactness of seat position in a group of riders, so it is impossible to achieve an exact outline in a number of different horses. The use of the various reins undoubtedly affects the position of head and neck, but they should never be used by a person who does not have effective legs, for the fore and hind ends of a horse must move in a synchronised fashion. Without effective legs it is impossible to ensure that hind quarter activity mirrors that of the forelimbs, dictated by the use of the various 'reins'.

To work on the forehand only, without correct engagement of hock and hind quarter muscle is a waste of valuable time, the horse will learn to go in a manner which achieves collection and activity in front, due to the enforced change of head and neck position, but with no impulsion from behind.

Running rein

William Cavendish, Duke of Newcastle (1592–1676) designed the running rein. It was commonly used throughout the period of classical training. The rein was fastened under the saddle flaps before returning via the bit rings to the rider's hands. The rein passed from the inside to the outside of the bit ring and was similar to the draw rein (see below). There is however a difference in the action of the two. The running rein causes the nose to be brought inward but places less emphasis on the lowering of the head, allowing the horse to balance its back in a manner to which it has become accustomed and is comfortable. The purpose of this rein is to increase the isometric toning activity of the muscles of the neck.

Draw rein

The draw rein, as its name suggests draws the head downwards, as well as causing the nose to be brought in towards the chest. The idea of the rein is to assist in shortening and to achieve a rounded outline.

The rein is fastened to the girth and, like the running rein, passes from the inner side of the bit ring to the outer and thence to the rider's hands. The running rein is rarely used today, but the draw rein has become common as people attempt to create an outline in many cases before the horse's musculature has been sufficiently prepared to achieve the required shape.

There are several possible results/problems to consider. Horses ridden continuously in draw reins, tend to become used to them, leaning upon the rein restraint in order to balance. Another problem is flexion. This tends to occur primarily at the joint between the head and first neck vertebra. It does not achieve effective nuchal ligament traction, as with generalised neck flexion, so the back loses support. With maximum flexion at this joint, the horse may also go behind the bit. As forward progression is one of the most important attributes of the well-trained horse, this is not helpful.

The balancing rein

This type of restraint was perfected by the late Major Peter Abbot Davis. It was vigorously promoted in the press and through public demonstrations given throughout the United Kingdom. The object of the balancing rein was to try to build the muscles of both back and neck in a relatively short space of time.

There are three ways of fitting the Abbot Davis balancing rein, the first is a straight attachment mouth to girth, the second from tail to mouth, the third from the mouth upwards. The design incorporates rubber sections which work as springs, with the angles of the straps employed acting as pulleys. It is a system which requires instruction from an expert to achieve success.

It is interesting to note that the use of a rein attached from the tail to the mouth can be seen in the carvings of the facade of the temple of Ramses III, when chariot horses were tail reined to counter both onesidedness and a lack of impulsion from behind. The principle behind the Abbot Davis is that the back is rounded and the quarters are actively brought under the body at the same time as the head and neck are lowered. The idea appears once again to be an attempted short cut in order to produce the outline.

The chambon

The chambon was designed to re-school animals which had adopted an unnaturally high head carriage and developed an upside-down neck, and was designed to be used on the lunge. Invented in France, this rein is rarely used in the UK, although common in many European training establishments and the subject of a book published in 1988 by J.A. Allen (Launder 1988).

The girth of saddle or roller acts as an anchorage for the strap, which passing upwards, splits, looking rather like an elongated running martingale. Each strap continues to the poll where each is threaded through a ring sited just below each ear, attached to either end of a padded cavesson headpiece. Each strap passes downwards, parallel with the bridle cheek pieces to be attached to the ring of a snaffle bit. The device, useful as it is, has little or no 'give' as has the latest rein based on similar principles.

The bungee rein

This is constructed from a single, strong rubber cord, shaped like an elongated U, the centre of which is passed through a moveable constrictor to afford length adjustment.

The centre of the U is placed at the poll, the two arms are passed down on either side of the cheek straps, through the snaffle rings and then continue downwards meeting at the girth where each dips to a centrally placed noose through which the firths have been passed. Adjustment for length is achieved by moving the constrictor ring on the cords at the poll.

The rein is very kind, encouraging flexion throughout the neck complex, so achieving the back lift necessary to allow hindquarter engagement.

The de Gogue

This rein was also developed in France. The de Gogue was designed to be used by experts to correct, when riding, problems at the poll, base of the neck or for a horse described as 'strong'. The cords, which in the chambon are attached to the bit, pass through the snaffle rings to continue as a rein allowing considerably more rider influence. As with all other aids the device was developed for use by experts rather than novice riders and although originally conceived to correct problems, a theory developed suggesting that usage built the muscles of the adopted position and that once those muscles had developed, the position would be retained automatically.

The reins are a method of increasing the resistance to the activity of muscle, thereby improving their competence, but the methodology employed by the reins does not imprint a brain response which will be generated automatically once the reins have been removed. This is because the horse needs the command, given by the rein, in order to activate the response.

If a horse is not going forward as it should, or adopting the positions required by the rider for its particular discipline, it is far better to go back to the beginning and start once again in long reins before resorting to highly sophisticated training aids designed by a 'master' of equitation. The bungee is probably the only exception to this.

24 The Addition of Skills

In any training regime, the long slow distance work (LSD) involves both the horse and the rider. The work undertaken is aimed at conditioning and improving muscle tone, while, at the same time the skeletal system of the horse begins its adaptive processes. At the end of this period, six weeks for older horses who have had a short 'holiday', eight to ten weeks for those returning to training after a long lay off and twelve weeks for youngsters starting their career, progressive muscle loading should be increased. During the LSD period, interspersed with being ridden out, some of the activities described under formal exercises can be incorporated both to add variety and to begin to include short lessons.

Riders, particularly novice riders, should try to incorporate the exercises suggested 'off horse' during the LSD period. Then as both horse and rider begin to tone their individual musculature, it is time to join the two together in a series of ridden gymnastic activities. As previously stated, all dancers, no matter what is to be their eventual dance discipline, start with the basic principles laid down by the exercises of the classical ballet school. No matter what is to be the eventual discipline of the riding horse, Thoroughbred racing horses excepted, the fundamental principles of the equine classical school provide an invaluable set of activities. The reason that classical work can be disadvantageous to the TB racehorse, is the fact that while for distance races endurance is necessary, the horse relies on natural stretch and recoil. Too much 'flat work' can change this, muscles having been trained in the middle, rather than outer range.

Nuno Oliveira said,

> 'the horse is not a machine, it is a living being one rides him and he never forgets the movements he has learned, but what the rider must remember is it is necessary to know and to always give the commands correctly, always return to basic exercises and spend time with them. The rider should be so sensitive that he can feel from the back of the horse and should know even if the horse has slept in a bad position in his stable'.

(Oliveira 1988)

The tactful rider feels if part of the horse is tired and knows how to engage this part and to change the forces to other areas. Oliveira also states that 'all riders must try to relax their hands and have a light contact'. In order to achieve light contact, a rider must have a seat independent of their hands.

As described above, ridden work over cavalletti is an excellent way of improving rider balance and is also an excellent way of increasing the loading for the horse, particularly if the animal has previously been being worked over cavalletti from the ground. A useful learning/improvement routine for both would be to work a horse in the arena with the cavalletti poles arranged down one long side at walk spacing and on the other long side at trot spacing.

All activity should begin with the horse ridden on a loose rein around the arena, then gradually achieving more collection. When the animal is warmed up and the rider begins to relax in the saddle, the horse is ridden down the line of walk-placed cavalletti, circles and is ridden down the trot-placed cavalletti. Both these activities should, if possible, occur on a loose rein in order that the horse balances itself, and becomes accustomed to carrying rider weight as it varies limb movements to step over the raised poles.

If the horse has been performing all the varied activities relatively readily and then, one day, seems unwilling to work, do not persist, take the animal out for a ride and try again another day. It may be that you, the rider, are not concentrating and are giving incorrect commands. The horse may have become thoroughly bored and for some reason is not going to make any effort.

When giving lessons (to the horse), the golden rule is practise in walk and get it right before progressing to trot, not only because you are trying to imprint a closed chain reflex, but also because the effort required both mentally and physically will be greater at trot than at walk. The progressive loading of the musculature continues by introducing canter to the horse's programme both in and out of the school. Progression from walk to canter achieves balance and suppleness. Start by changing from collected trot to canter then down to collected trot before attempting walk to canter. When the attempt to change from walk to canter is made, make certain that the horse is on a circle, then when on the circle in a corner, apply the aids for canter. It is essential that the horse learns to move into a canter smoothly.

Progressive loading, ridden work over cavalletti and simple classical exercises, should all continue to be included in general training until the suppleness and obedience required for the eventual task have been achieved. The length of time it will take for this to occur will vary with each horse and will depend on its early training, its muscle capability, its learning ability and its attitude.

There is a reason for going back to the basics even with a newly acquired old horse, because the horse, while it may have learned some of the movements required, has to learn a set of slightly new commands from each rider. It is extremely difficult for a horse to be trained and schooled by one person and then ridden by another. Great riders are in tune with their horses and able to ride apparently any horse without previous experience of the animal. Notables today in the UK would be Frankie Dettori, flat-race jockey, A.P. Macoy and Richard Johnson, National Hunt jump jockeys, William Fox-Pitt, and Andrew Nicholson, three-day eventing, Carl Hester, dressage, and the Wittaker family from among the show-jumping fraternity.

Adequate exposure to competition requirements

No matter what the eventual level of excellence or competition requirement, exposure to all expected demands pre-competition is essential, not only for success but also to avoid, as far as it possible, injury by pre-conditioning tissues. Horses trained, for example for endurance in flat areas, suddenly meeting the heather-covered slopes of Exmoor are rather like skiers who have never experienced powder snow – confused and off balance. It is therefore sensible for the rider and trainer to have understood fully, by attending events before competing, the requirements of that competition.

One of the more difficult things for a horse to do is to jump downhill, when a considerable amount of eccentric work is demanded. Muscles and tendons can learn what is expected in this situation but only after gradual exposure to the activity. If you wish to teach your horse to jump downhill, start over small obstacles on easy inclines, and gradually increase the size of the fence. Then find an incline with a steeper angle, and use the same procedure, small fence first then gradually make the task more difficult. Do not attempt any new activity more than four or five times at each session, muscles and all soft tissues tire easily when exposed to new tasks.

Many of the training areas attached to French racing centres are sited in wooded areas. There are countless trails through the woods, which are on hills, nearly all the tracks sport fences of different types and heights, allowing riders to trot, canter and gallop their animals over a variety of obstacles. Fences are also sited on uphill and downhill slopes. Jumps into water are another hazard requiring a huge learning curve and a great deal of practice. Have you ever jumped into water and tried to run? It is often possible with the co-operation of local landowners, to create similar training conditions to those enjoyed in France.

Once the basic learning has been experienced, balance and co-ordination trained, the patterns become a cortical imprint. No experience will ever mirror competition exactly, but remember, few outdoor competitions be they endurance, showing, jumping or event, take place on manicured, flat surfaces such as are found in the 'all weather' arena or on the 'all weather' track. There is little point in preparing in perfect conditions then having to compete on a rough, probably undulating or sloping surface. Natural horses in the wild, animals turned away on moors, on bogs, hills or mountains are all far more balanced than those living in flat level conditions. As sure footed as a mountain pony is a pertinent saying.

Further reading

Launder, E. & Legard, H. *Understanding The Chambon*, J.A. Allen, London, 1988

Oliveira, N. *Classical Principles of the Art of Training Horses*, Howley and Russell, Australia, 1988

Tellington-Jones, L. *Improve Your Horse's Well-Being*, Trafalgar Square Publishing, Vermont, USA, 1999

General Summary

25 The Fundamentals of Natural Training and Husbandry

The Nature of Horses by Stephen Budianski (1997) should be the starting point for all who wish to embrace natural horsemanship. This should be followed by consideration of the principles of Monty Roberts and allied to those of the past masters of equitation, starting with Xenophon (371 BC).

Many books are written about the management of the horse and its presumed thought processes and while some consider that domestication must have endowed the horse with human concepts, it has in fact developed along a different evolutionary path from man – one which requires it to be able to get up and run within minutes of birth.

It is worth considering the following points:

- The hairs of a horse's coat are designed regulate its body temperature (we cut them off);
- Its nasal whiskers inform the animal if there is space for its head in a narrow area (we cut them off);
- The horse was not really designed for carrying a rider (saddle design should necessitate comfort for the horse rather than the rider);
- The animal has a digestive system designed to achieve nutritional requirements from continual browsing, to trickle feed, rather than have set amounts of feed two or three times a day.

Amazingly enough, the horse survives the many human foibles considered to be in its best interests. To carry man, without detriment to itself, it must be trained. There are no short cuts to fitness and no therapies or aids which are going to improve the animal's capabilities without regular exercise.

Just as with human athletes, all horses have a level of achievement which may be constrained by a number of features. The first of these is conformation. Some horses are unable to perform some tasks because their conformation does not allow them to execute certain movements. The second is their mental attitude. Horses which have been damaged mentally at some time in their career, have suffered a considerable amount of pain, or have become bored and dissatisfied will be very, very, difficult to change. This sort of animal needs a total change of venue and training programme. It is particularly important to remember this if trying to change a lifestyle from domestic to natural living. It is a shock to the horse's system to change from being in a stable, rugged up, fed twice or three times daily, to being turned out in a field.

Always bear in mind that:

- horses' bodies adapt best when exposed to small, regular increases in exercise (progressive loading);
- unless progressive loading is achieved, the response to training will be negligible;
- any increase, too fast or too strenuous can produce unwanted results, including tissue damage;

- muscles respond quite rapidly to loading and exercise but other tissues – bone, ligaments, tendons, joints and the feet – take time;
- you are not training one single structure, you are training a complicated interaction of systems;
- never neglect the endurance-type long, slow building work;
- the speed of an activity and the distance that the horse must cover are two separate entities;
- as the training programme develops, develop speed independent of distance;
- physical and physiological effects are not instant and the result of training will not show for three or four days after an increase in work. A horse may respond to a sharp bout of interval training on the day in question, but three days later be dull and unable to perform simple tasks, this indicates progression has been rushed.

Remember that response to training slows with ageing. Never forget that each horse, just like each person, is an individual and will respond in a slightly different manner from others in your stable or stabled in the same yard. It is of course perfectly possible to ride a horse from the field or from the stable without any attempt at improving its physical fitness and many horses do survive in this manner. However, if you wish to compete, to enjoy your horse and want your horse to enjoy you, it is sensible to build in some form of athletic training programme. People have been doing this in Europe years, whereas the British tended to regard the Classical School and European teachings as 'foppish'. Traditionally to the British, riding was not an art, the horse was a means of transport, an agricultural necessity, or to be ridden for pleasure or for racing. No one built riding schools as they did in Europe.

Today's scientific knowledge and the inclusion of scientific principles have allowed horsemen to achieve feats of excellence with their mounts. However, when we consider the conquests by Alexander the Great, even Napoleon, it is as well to pause and to wonder if today's feats really are a first, or if the horse after World War I just took a back seat, making way for the early excitement created by the motor car and we are merely, as the twenty-first century emerges, rediscovering its amazing versatility.

Appendix I

Programme Design

Many people, especially those newly introduced to horses, find it difficult to understand that there are no definite, written recipes for training as there are for cooking. Training is an art, to be successful you have to understand the effects of the varied activities called exercises. You should then be able to select a combination best suited to the individual requirements of yourself and the animal in question.

First considerations

Horse	age
	conformation
	previous experiences
	current level of fitness
	previous problems
Rider	expectations
	experience/training, riding expertise
	time available
	own fitness
Facilities	local hacking facilities
	school/arena
	gymnastic apparatus (poles, fences)
End requirement	levels of competition aimed for
	spacing between competitions
	specialist requirements

Work and lessons

When planning a training programme it is essential to understand the difference between *work* and *lessons*.

Work develops the horse's strength, improves cardiovascular efficiency and prepares the animal for lessons.

Lessons involve obedience, gradually learnt by the horse. During lessons the horse learns to respond and perform to rider command and by so doing, eventually to execute the movements or perform the activities required by the rider in response to the aids. Lessons follow work, the work having settled the horse before asking it for concentration and full attention. The time allocated for each individual lesson should be short, the horse has a small attention span and endless repetition 'to try to get it right' will cause fatigue, boredom, even resentment, depending on the temperament of the individual animal.

It is advisable, if the horse keeps making mistakes or fails to learn or perfect a new activity, to change the lesson, returning to try again later. In this case the rider or trainer should reflect on their input. Were the commands clear? Was the horse correctly balanced? *Who went wrong, horse or trainer?*

Muddled signals make it difficult for the horse to respond correctly; a comparison is like a person trying to understand the instructions for setting a new watch, if those instructions are in Russian and the purchaser can only read English. *Lessons* should be interspersed throughout the *work* programme.

The following points are useful when considering designing a programme:

- Work from the ground first in long reins. Then, when the horse has conditioned the base musculature, a lunge is excellent for both correction of faults and the building of postural and activity muscle groups.
- Periods of long, slow distance work must be incorporated into the final work programme following its use in early preparation.
- Riding out across fields, over commons or park land, in woods, across moorland, in hill or mountain country keeps both horse and rider alert and entertained. It also improves balance in both horse and rider, improves co-ordination between rider and horse, and improves reflex responses in all the joints of both. Vary the activities when on a ride. If there is an even stretch with a useful hedge, practice for example, a shoulder in, change pace, incorporate variety. In Sweden this type of riding is called 'speed play', as previously discussed.

Over recent years, training has tended to become stereotyped and far too regulated. Lighten it. Even if you do not incorporate scientific interval training within the general programme, by monitoring the heart rate and its return to normal you will have a good indication of the level of fitness achieved.

When you are satisfied that the horse is ready to compete start with small local events, preferably those that will mimic the eventual demands of your discipline. For example, endurance riders might consider taking part in a sponsored ten-mile ride, horses could jump at clear round events at local riding clubs, event horses could take part in hunter trials, dressage horses and event horses should compete at small, non-taxing competitions. Make these experiences pleasant and mentally stressless for your horse by not asking too much of it.

Make these outings a self-learning curve. There is no need to panic if a vital girth has been left behind, it will not happen a second time and it is better to make mistakes when it is not an important event rather than at the first serious competition, for a disciplined approach is as essential for rider as it is for the horse.

Appendix II

Athletic Horse Versus Athletic Man

The studies show that in athletic terms, the horse is superior to man. The physiological changes resulting from heavy exercise have been assessed in both species, demonstrating the following variations:

- muscle tissue accounts for 41% of body mass in the horse, 45% in man;
- respiratory exchange in the horse under exercise conditions is nearly twice that of man;
- the cardiac output in the horse under exercise conditions and calculated per kg of body weight is twice that of man;
- during exercise the concentration of circulating haemoglobin doubles in the horse, there is a scarcely perceptible increase in man.

These findings show that the interaction between the spleen, heart and muscles in the horse is more efficient than in man due to:

1. a higher concentration of arterial oxygen;
2. a greater cardiac output;
3. a more efficient extraction of oxygen during activity;
4. although subject to similar 'waste' during activity, the horse appears able to:
    a. tolerate higher blood lactate levels than man;
    b. still maintain a lower pH than man;
    c. tolerate increased acidosis;
    d. has a greater capacity to buffer (resist) acid/alkali changes.

A feature common to both horse and man appears to be that both species demonstrate inadequate lung function. In the horse, this may be secondary to the effects of rider weight and the effect of the girth.

The horse demonstrates a physiological activity potential superior to man but an inability to achieve the potential, *possibly* due to impaired respiratory ability. Exercise tolerance studies suggest that the horse would be superior if adequate oxygen were available. Only a few physiological variations have been isolated through research, but there would appear to be sufficient evidence to suggest that concepts associated with human athletic performance may well not be pertinent to the horse. The human model for example has a preconceived idea of requirement, both during training and at competition. Before running a marathon a participant will decide what to eat the previous day and how long he or she needs to warm up. The human athlete has the ability to *decide* his or her course of action and a brain allowing him or her to think and plan ahead. Not only must the horse do exactly what it is commanded by the rider but it has *no idea*, when travelling for example, how long the journey will be, what lies in store at the other end or the tasks it will be expected to undertake. There is no way a horse can preconceive and prepare. Man prepares mentally, how can the horse do so? In effect, there are two species to train, the art is to prepare both, then join them to perform as a team.

Appendix III

Natural Health Maintenance in The New-Age Horse

Stabling

If stabled, keep the top door of the loose box open at all times, increasing the number of rugs to maintain warmth. Make certain there is adequate airflow through the stable but not cold drafts.

Bedding

Mats are a great boon if the floor drains.

Shavings

If they are damp or slightly dusty, then you need to change your supplier. Sweep walls/ledges regularly while the horse is out of the box to remove any residual dust.

Paper bedding

Print dust is a chemical hazard arising from poor quality newsprint. If you find a fine, grey-black dust on walls or ledges, you have a chemical dust problem. Dampen or change the bedding.

Straw bedding

Avoid dusty, short straw. Shake up the bed with the horse out of the box. Remember to ask if the crop from which the straw came was sprayed with chemicals. Use organic straw whenever possible.

Rugs

Shake daily outside the box and away from the horse.

Grooming

Groom in a well-ventilated area, outside if possible. Why pollute the horse's box with its dust, leaving particles suspended in the air for the animal or you to inhale while you are grooming?

Hay

Shake up the hay in a well-ventilated area and shake just before feeding. Dust shaken out of the hay will sink back on to it, if the hay is beneath its own dust cloud.

Always check for mould. *DO NOT USE MOULDY HAY OR HAYLAGE-TYPE FODDER WHICH IS FERMENTING.*

Ask for an analysis of the hay. Protein levels in the hay are important. If there are high protein levels in your hay or haylage cut down hard food levels.

Disinfectants

Remember that all disinfectants, like chemical sprays, must kill in order to be effective. Their purpose is to destroy harmful life forms, ensure that the local environment is rendered 'unfriendly' to those life forms and so avoid a reproduction of those life forms. The sprays and disinfectants are designed to lose their toxicity after a period of stated time. Do not ignore the time periods stated.

If you spray a box wearing a mask and then put a horse into the area before the spray has detoxified the horse will inhale the toxin.

Chemical sprays

Avoid riding through any area which has recently been sprayed, particularly if it has not rained since spraying commenced. Avoid any area where aerial spraying is in process. Avoid any area where sheep have been dipped – dips are dangerous. If spraying your own land or yard, read and follow the instructions, they are printed for very good reasons. All chemicals in excess are toxic to varying degrees.

Oil seed rape

Oil seed rape is a member of the brassica (cabbage) family. After flowering, this plant group produces certain chemicals. Rape produces large quantities of natural insecticides, sulphur-containing volatile chemicals including benzyl and phenolaldehydes. In some cases these trigger allergic reactions similar to hay fever (Hanlon 2008).

Indoor arenas

All indoor arenas should have a sprinkler system. If dust is seen on any surface, it has come from somewhere. It may have been thrown into the air by horses working on the surface, eventually settling. If dust is there to settle, then it is there in the air to inhale.

Lay the dust and increase the ventilation by all means possible. Watering increases part-icle weight, reducing the height of particle movement.

All-weather surfaces

There is a kick back of fine particles at speed on this surface no matter what the manu-facturers claim. On all-weather gallops jockeys wear goggles to protect their eye, *horses are inhaling the dust the jockeys are experiencing.* All-weather surfaces *must* be main-tained to the standards advocated by the manufacturers, this will reduce the likelihood of particle inhalation but *will not* totally remove it.

Travelling horses

Horse boxes and trailers should be well ventilated. Remember that as a moving vehicle cuts through the air and deflects it sideways, a vacuum is created at its rear, suction then pulls air into the box from behind the transport. This air is usually chemically polluted by exhaust fumes. Horses lucky enough to be near an open window press their noses to the gap trying to breathe fresh air from outside the box.

Remember the horse, while travelling, is working to balance for the entire journey, the muscle work requires oxygen. Four horses in a lorry use a lot of air and expel an awful lot of waste. Leardon (Irish Equine Research) has shown that most horses travel in a chemically polluted air situation and that the levels of pollution enhance the ability of various bacteria and micro-organisms to reproduce, reaching a level which constitutes an infectious dosage in a very short time.

Man is free to both choose and change his environment. If a room is stuffy, man opens a window, if the car inhales foul air through the heating system man opens a window to change the air. The domestic horse is forced to endure conditions created by man, he cannot control the ventilation of his stable or of his transport, a great deal of lung dam-age occurs as a result of thoughtlessness on the part of the horse carer. Remember, that the lungs of both man and equine are very delicate, they need consideration and care.

Further reading

Hanlon, M. 'Be Wary of the Yellow Peril', *Western Morning News*, 20/05/2008

Glossary

Abdomen: the part of the body which lies between the chest and the pelvis

Abduction: a drawing away from the median plane of the body

Absorption: the uptake of substances into or across tissues

Acupuncture: Chinese science of influencing the body systems

Adduction: a drawing towards the median plane of the body

Aerobic: functions which can only occur in the presence of an oxygen molecule

Amino acid: the body proteins necessary for all functions are composed of amino acids; some are manufactured by the body, others are extracted from food

Anaerobic: function which occurs in the absence of oxygen

Anion: an ion which conducts negatively charged electricity

Anterior: situated in front of, or in the forward part of, an organ; towards the head end of the body

Arteriole: a very small branch of the arterial system connecting to a capillary

Artery: a blood vessel containing arterial blood charged with cells, oxygen and fuel. Arteries are sited to allow the passage of blood away from the heart

Atrophy: wasting away of a normally developed organ or tissue due to degeneration of cells

Avascular: not supplied with blood vessels

Avulsion: the tearing away of part of a structure

Balance: (Chinese concept) the necessity for harmony within all systems of living organisms

Bifurcation: the site where a single structure divides into two branches

Bilateral: prefix 'bi' relates to two, thus bilateral denotes both lateral sides

Blood pressure: the pressure of blood on the walls of the arteries, dependent on the energy of the heart action, the elasticity of the walls of the arteries, and the volume and viscosity of the blood

Bone: a dense connective tissue which forms the skeleton

Bone marrow: the internal cavities of the bones which act as factories manufacturing cells

Bronchus, bronchi: either or both of the two main branches of the trachea, one going to each lung

Bursa: a sac or sac-like cavity filled with fluid and situated at places in the tissues at which friction would otherwise develop

Bursitis: an inflammation of the bursa, occasionally accompanied by the formation of a calcific deposit in the underlying tendon

Capillary: a minute blood vessel, with walls only one cell thick, enabling the exchange of all components within the body's structures; the blood in the network is delivered by the arterioles and removed by the venules

Capsule: the tissue surrounding a joint and assisting in joint lubrication

Cardiac: pertaining to the heart

Cardiac cycle: the actions of the heart during one complete heart beat

Cartilage: a dense connective tissue

Catalyst: a substance capable of changing a chemical reaction and yet itself remaining unchanged

Cation: an ion which conducts positively charged electricity

Caudal: the area behind the central area of the horse's body

Cell: cells are the basic units of all life; all living organisms are composed of cells, each cell type is specialised and performs a particular function

Chelate: the process by which the body renders minerals usable

Ch'i: Chinese term for energy

Chronic: long-term, continued; not acute

Conformation: the shape or contour of the body or body structures

Congenital: existing at and usually before birth; referring to conditions which may or may not be inherited

Connective tissue: tissue which binds other tissues together into functional units. Variations in the composition of the basic elements give rise to a variety of functional differences

Contusion: a bruise or injury incurred without breaking the skin

Cranium: the bones enclosing and protecting the brain, *adj. Cranial*

Diagnosis: identifying a disease from its characteristics and/or causative agent; distinguishing one disease from another

Diaphragm: the muscular membrane separating the abdominal and chest cavities

Dilatation: the condition of being dilated or stretched beyond normal dimensions

Dilation: a stretching or expansion

Dislocation: the displacement of any part, usually referring to a bone

Distal: a point further from the centre of the body

Distension: the state of being swollen or enlarged from internal pressure

Dorsal: pertaining to the back or denoting a position more towards the back surface than some other point of reference

DNA: genetic material present in all cells

Dynamisation: a process in the preparation of homoeopathic remedies

Dysfunction: disturbance or impairing of the function of an organ

Electrolyte: a single, pure chemical substance capable of carrying either a positive or negative charge. Electrolytes are lost in urine, by excessive sweating and diarrhoea. When levels of electrolytes are severely diminished, they need to be replaced by giving the appropriate substance via the mouth or by intravenous drip

Enzyme: the catalyst of a biochemical reaction

Epidermis: the outermost layer of skin, not supplied with blood vessels

Epithelium: the covering of internal and external surfaces of the body, including the lining of vessels and other small cavities; it consists of cells joined together by small amounts of cementing substances

Excretion: the removal of metabolic waste from the body

Extension: a movement which brings a limb into a straight line

Extensor: any muscle which extends a joint

Extracellular: outside the confines of the cells

Fascia: a connective tissue found throughout the body

Fen: a Chinese measurement: 10 *fen* = 1 *tsun*

Fibrosis: the formation of fibrous tissue

Flexion: the act of bending

Fossa: a hollow or depressed area

Haematoma: an accumulation of blood within the tissues which clots to form a solid swelling

Haemoglobin: the oxygen-carrying protein pigment of the red blood cells

Haemorrhage: the escape of blood from the vessels; bleeding

Hyperextension: extreme or excessive extension of a limb

Hyperflexion: forced overflexion of a limb or a part of a limb

Hypersensitivity: a state of altered activity in which the body reacts with an exaggerated response to a foreign agent

Insertion: the point of attachment of a muscle (e.g. to a bone)

Inspiration: the act of inhaling or drawing air into the lungs

Intracellular: interactions taking place with a cell

Intravenous: within a vein

Involuntary: performed independently of the will

Ion: an electrically charged particle

Ischaemia: inadequate circulatory flow caused by constriction of the local blood vessels

Joint: the place of union or junction between two or more bones of the skeleton

Larynx: the structure of muscle and cartilage located at the top of the trachea and below the root of the tongue; the 'voice box'

Lateral: pertaining to a side or outer surface; a position further from the midline of the body or of a structure

Ligament: a band of fibrous tissue which connects bones or cartilages

Lumbar: pertaining to the loins, the part of the back between the thorax and pelvis

Lymph: a transparent, yellowish liquid containing mostly white blood cells and derived from tissue fluids

Medial: pertaining to the middle or inner surface; a position closer to the midline of the body or of a structure

Meridians: conceptual paths within the body considered by the Chinese to interlink all body organs

Mobility: the ability to move

Mother tincture: a term used to denote the source of a remedy in the Bach Flower remedies

Muscle: tissue which by contraction produces movement

Muscle tremor: an involuntary trembling or quivering of a muscle

Necrosis: death of a cell or group of cells

Nerves: fibres which convey impulses between a part of the central nervous system and some other region of the body

Non-vascular: not supplied with blood vessels

Nosode: material extracted from the product of a condition or disease and used to effect a cure

Oedema: excessive accumulation of fluid in the body tissues

Optic: pertaining to the eye

Ossify: to change or develop into bone

Palpation: the act of feeling with the hand

Periostium: outer covering of a bone

Plasma: the liquid portion of the blood, containing the suspended components

Platelets: disc-shaped structures found in the blood of all mammals and chiefly known for their role in the blood coagulation: also called *blood platelets*. (See also *Thrombocytes*)

Plexus: a network of lymphatic vessels, nerves, veins or arteries

Point: the term used to describe the area where acupressure or acupuncture should be administered

Posterior: situated behind, or in the back of, a structure; towards the rear end of the body

Potency: required dilution of a homoeopathic remedy

Prognosis: the prospect of recovery from a disease or injury

Progressive: advancing, going from bad to worse; advancing in severity

Proud flesh: excessive granulation tissue

Pulmonary: pertaining to the lungs

Pulse: rhythmic throbbing of an artery which may be felt with the finger; caused by blood forced through the vessel as a result of contractions of the heart

Red blood cells: haemoglobin-carrying corpuscles in the blood, which transport oxygen

Regeneration: the natural renewal of a structure following damage

Remedy: the term used in homoeopathy to describe the appropriate restorative for a diagnosed problem

RNA: concerned with protein synthesis

Rotation: the process of turning around an axis

Scar tissue: tissue remaining after the healing of a wound or other morbid process

Septum: a dividing wall or partition

Subacute: somewhat acute, between acute and chronic

Subluxation: an incomplete or partial dislocation

Succussion: a process of shaking, essential in the preparation of homoeopathic remedies

Supraspinous: above a spine or spinous process

Thrombocytes: blood platelets

Tsun: a Chinese term for measurement (see also *Fen*)

Vein: a vessel through which the blood passes from various organs or parts, back to the heart

Venous: pertaining to the veins

Virus: a particle which uses cells as a host and replicates within chosen cells; the effects of the replication are toxic and cause side effects toxic to the main host. Vaccines do control some viral invasions, antibiotics are ineffective against viruses but may be needed to control secondary infections

Voluntary: in accordance with the will

Yang: Chinese term for positive energy

Yin: Chinese term for negative energy

General Bibliography

Baucher, F. *A Method of Horsemanship Founded Upon New Principles*, Kessinger, US, 2006

Becher, R. *Schooling by the Natural Method*, 1963 (out of print)

Berens von Rautenfeld, D. *Manuelle Lymphdrainage beim Pferd*, Schlutersche VCh Erlagasgesellschaft mbH & Co.

Budianski, S. *The Nature of Horses*, Phoenix Orion, London, 1997

Burger, U. & Zietzschmann, O. *The Rider Forms the Horse*, FN Verlag, Warendorf, Germany, 2003

Clayton, H.M. *Conditioning Sport Horses*, Sport Horse Publications, Saskatoon, 1991 (out of print)

Cook, W.R. *Specifications for Speed in the Racehorse*, Russell Meerdink Co Ltd, USA, 1989

Davies, B., Eagle, D., Finney, B., *Soil Management*, 5th edn, Farming Press, Ipswich, UK, 1993

Decarpentry, General, (trans. Bartle, N.) *Academic Education*, J.A. Allen, 2001

Denoix, J.M. *Biomécanique et Travail Physique du Cheval*. RCS Versailles, Paris, 1992

Denoix, J.M. & Pailloux, J.P. *Approche du Kinesithérapie du Cheval*, Maloine, Paris, 1997

Dumas, E. *The Horses of the Sahara*, University of Texas Press, Austin, US, 1986

Gawani Ponyboy, *Out of the Saddle: Native American Horsemanship*, Bow Tie Press, Irvine California, 1998

Giniaux, D. *Soulagez Votre Cheval aux Doigts*, Favre, Paris, 1993

Hartley-Edwards, E. *Training Aids in Theory and Practice*, J.A. Allen, London, 1990

Heuschmann, G. *Tug of War: Classical versus Modern Dressage*, J.A. Allen, London, 2007

Johnson, A.M. *Equine Medical Disorders*, 2nd edn, Blackwell Scientific Publications, Oxford, 1994

Jones, W.E. *Equine Sports Medicine*, Lea and Febiger, USA, 1989

Karl, P. *Long Reining – The Saumur Method*, J.A. Allen, London, 2003

Kellon, E.M. *Equine Supplements and Nutraceuticals*, Breakthrough Publications, Ossining, NY, 1998

Kyrklund, K. *Dressage with Kyra*, Kenilworth Press, 2006

Marks, K. *Perfect Confidence*, Ebury Press, 2007

Marks, K. *Perfect Manners*, Ebury Press, 2002 (see also: www.intelligenthorsemanship. co.uk)

Oliveira, N. *Classical Principles of the Art of Training Horses*, Howley & Russell, Australia, 1983

Podhaisky, A., (trans. V.D.S. Williams), *The Complete Training of Horse and Rider*, Harrap & Co. London, 1967

Roberts, M. *Ask Monty*, Headline, London, 2007

Roberts, M. *The Man Who Listens to Horses*, Arrow Books, London, 1997

Rooney, J.R. *The Mechanics of the Horse*, Krieger, New York, 1981

Snow, D.H. & Vogel, C.J. *Equine Fitness*, David and Charles, Newton Abbot, Devon, 1987

Stanier, S. *The Art of Lungeing*, J.A. Allen, London, 1993

Stanier, S. *The Art of Long Reining*, J.A. Allen, London, 1993

Steinbrecht, G. *The Gymnasium of the Horse*, Xenophon Press, Cleveland, Ohio, 1995

Stodulka, R. *Medizinische Reitlehrer*, Parey, Stuttgart, 2006

Xenophon, (circa 450 BC) *The Art of Horsemanship* (trans. M.H. Morgan), J.A. Allen, London, 1993

Useful Addresses

Including suppliers of natural products

National Institute of Medical Herbalists
Elm House
54 Mary Arches Street
Exeter EX4 3BA
Tel: 01392 426022
Fax: 01392 498963
Email: nimh@ukexeter.freeserve.co.uk
Website: http://www.nimh.org.uk

School of Phytotherapy (Herbal Medicine)
Bucksteep Manor
Bodle Street Green
Near Hailsham
East Sussex BN27 4RJ
Tel: 01323 834800
Email: medherb@pavilion.co.uk

British Association of Homoeopathic Veterinary Surgeons (BAHVS)
The Veterinary Dean
The Faculty of Homoeopathy
2 Powis Place
Great Ormond Street
London WC1N 3HT
Email: enquiries@bahvs.com
Website: http://www.bahvs.com

The British Homoeopathic Association
Hahnemann House
29 Park Street West
Luton LU1 3BE
Tel: 0870 444 3950
Fax: 0870 444 3960
Website: www.trusthomeopathy.org

Ainsworths Homoeopathic Pharmacy
34 New Cavendish Street
London W1G 8UF
Tel: 020 7935 5330

Hair and soil analysis
Thompson and Joseph
T & J House
119 Plumstead Road
Norwich NR1 4JT

Leech farm
Bryngwili Road
Hendy
Carmarthenshire SA4 0XT
Website: www.biopharm-leeches.com

Camrosa Equestrian Ltd: www.camrosa.co.uk

Eustace: www.laminitisclinic.com

Equine America: www.equine-america.co.uk

Equine Health Center Ltd: www.equinehealthcenter.com

Hilton Herbs: www.hiltonherbssusa.com.

Horsefair Equestrian International: www.horsefair.co.uk

Holistic Horse: pat@holistichorse.com

Botanical animal flower essences: Stacey@equilite.com (USA)

Intelligent Horsemanship Association: www.intelligenthorsemanship.co.uk

The Stable Collection (pure plant oil production): www.susangeorgenaturally.com

Index

Printed and bound by CPI Group (UK) Ltd, Croydon, CR0 4YY